❧ Relief, Naturally ❧

Did you know:

- ❀ raw natural honey can soothe the pain of mild burns?
- ❀ certain potatoes relieve skin irritation and itching?
- ❀ castor oil can help the body reabsorb cysts?
- ❀ sage leaf tea or tea tree oil can solve dandruff problems?
- ❀ sprinkling powdered ginger into your children's mittens and socks will keep their extremities toasty while playing outdoors?
- ❀ raspberry leaf is a marvelous all-around tonic that bolsters the immune system?

Whether your children are suffering from teething pains, asthma, diarrhea, insect bites, sunburn, a nosebleed, poison ivy, swollen glands, pink eye, chicken pox, constipation, a cold, or the flu, you'll find effective, practical solutions for their ailments in

GENTLE HEALING FOR BABY AND CHILD

Gentle Healing for Baby and Child

*A Parent's Guide
to Child-Friendly Herbs
and Other Natural Remedies for
Common Ailments and Injuries*

ANDREA CANDEE, MH, MSC
with
DAVID ANDRUSIA

POCKET BOOKS
New York London Toronto Sydney Singapore

POCKET BOOKS, a division of Simon & Schuster, Inc.
1230 Avenue of the Americas
New York, NY 10020

POCKET and colophon are registered trademarks of
Simon & Schuster, Inc.

Cover design by Anna Dorfman
Photo credits: Index Stock Photography, Eyewire, Zephyr Images, FoodPix

Printed in the United States of America

The authors of this book are not physicians and the ideas, procedures, and suggestions in this book are not intended as a substitute for the medical advice of a trained health professional. All matters regarding your child's health require medical supervision. Consult a physician before adopting the suggestions in this book, as well as about any condition that may require diagnosis or medical attention. In addition, the statements made by the authors regarding certain products and services represent the views of the authors alone, and do not constitute a recommendation or endorsement of any product or service by the publisher. While natural remedies are generally safe, it is not possible to predict an individual's reaction to a particular treatment or therapy. The authors and publisher disclaim any liability arising directly or indirectly from the use of the book, or of any products mentioned herein.

An *Original* Publication of POCKET BOOKS

10 9 8 7 6 5 4 3 2 1

Library of Congress Cataloging-In-Publication Data

Candee, Andrea.
    Gentle healing for baby and child : a parent's guide / Andrea Candee and David Andrusia.
        p.   cm.
    Includes bibliographical references.
    ISBN 978-0-7434-9725-1
    1. Herbs—Therapeutic use. 2. Pediatrics—Formulae, receipts, prescriptions. 3. Children—Diseases—Alternative treatment. I. Andrusia, David. II. Title.

RJ53.H47 C36 2000
615.5'42—dc21   00-060657

First Pocket Books trade paperback printing May 2001

For information regarding the special discounts for bulk purchases, please contact Simon & Schuster Special Sales at 1-800-456-6798 or business@simonandschuster.com

To my sons, Chris and Brian,
for being my loving, living experiments

And for taking an interest in who I am, not only as their mother,
but as a work in progress

❧ ❧

*You ought not to attempt to cure the eyes without the head
or the head without the body.*

*Neither ought you to attempt to cure the body without the soul.
For the part can never be well unless the whole is well.*
— SOCRATES

❧ Acknowledgments ❧

The development of this book has ridden on the encouragement of many wonderful supporters: my family, friends, professional associates, and clients.

❧ Special Thanks ❧

❧ to David Andrusia, for his talent in helping me to express my vision;

❧ to my editor, Emily Bestler, for her belief in the importance of this material and for her comments not only as an editor, but as a mother of small children as well;

❧ to Kip Hakala, assistant editor, whose enthusiasm prevailed;

❧ to Maury Hill, Jr., my loving, patient computer angel who never says "can't";

❧ to my mother, Lyla Soikin, for developing in me the self-confidence to know I can do anything, and for her wholehearted encouragement to make it happen;

❧ to my father, Bernard Soikin, although he no longer walks among us, his loving presence and support is with me always; and

❧ to Robert DeGaetano, who has championed my soul's growth with his unconditional love.

❧ Contents ❧

❧ Foreword ☙

Most textbooks of medicine have a peculiar disclaimer tucked away just before the opening pages. "The practice of medicine is ever-changing." Or, "Medical science is an evolving discipline. New discoveries are made every year." Then follows a warning to consider information presented and treatments declared in the context of when it was written and in light of newer, possibly more relevant data. This has been and certainly always will be true as scientists attempt to understand the roots of human suffering and healers seek to alleviate it.

Ten years ago, medical prognosticators may have foreseen some of the advances that define present day medical practice: computerized diagnostic and information systems, new antibiotics and vaccines, possibly even cloning, although that prediction would have been made by writers or readers of science fiction. But I don't believe that anyone, even a few years ago, would have stated seriously that the PDR (*Physician's Desk Reference*) would publish a compendium of herbal medicine products; or that the *Journal of the American Medical Association* would devote an entire issue to Complementary Medicine. Alternative medicine is not quite so "alternative" these days.

There is no alternative to competent, compassionate medical care. And that is why in a conventional pediatric practice we use alternative therapeutics. While modern medicine continues to perform miracles on a daily basis—organ transplantation, anti-cancer protocols, new vaccines—little progress has been made or even attention given to the minor (and not so minor) ailments that continue to plague humanity—the common cold, headaches, behavioral issues. We found that, in the case of ear infections, sometimes the prescribed medicines created other problems and occasionally didn't even cure. Finding effective alternatives to antibiotics is not so easy—one child's panacea may be another's placebo.

Enter Andrea Candee. She accepted immediately the invitation of two M.D.s and came to our office to teach us how to use herbs for a variety of pediatric complaints. We have had the opportunity to observe how effective, gentle, and well tolerated these remedies are in children. The information contained in this book is literally priceless. We use herbs daily in our practice and we use them with confidence when we treat our patients and our families.

Nurturing an ailing individual back to health is a gratifying experience that is shared by patient and healer. This book will show you how to do it. If you follow the advice in this book and take the time to search out the various herbal medicines that Ms. Candee recommends, I believe that you will discover that your children will get better quicker. The earlier in the course of an illness you intervene with an effective remedy, the less severe and prolonged the symptoms. And you might just find that a visit to the doctor is not necessary!

Larry Baskind, M.D., F.A.A.P.
Riverside Pediatrics
Croton on Hudson, New York

1

A Word from the Author

Today, according to the esteemed *Journal of the American Medical Association*, a full 42% of Americans have used natural healing therapies. To me, this is extremely good news because this was not always the case!

Although it was nearly 20 years ago, I vividly recall the afternoon I nervously gave my first talk on herbs to the local PTA. Even though I was among friends in a progressive community, I had no idea how they would react to my unconventional presentation on the healing power of herbs for children.

This was long before the popularity of Dr. Andrew Weil, organic foods, and the acknowledgment of the mind/body healing connection by the medical establishment. Keep in mind that until recently, "alternative" meant odd, and in many places in this country sprinkling sprouts on a salad was considered absolutely anti-establishment!

I was a mother of two sons and played an active role in the life of my town, so I felt people were willing to listen to what I had to say. My audience turned out to be receptive (albeit cautious) and I was encouraged to move forward with what was to become my life's work: sharing my knowledge of the healing power of herbs—at first with family and friends, then with clients—and now, with you.

Though I was devoted to my subject, I could hardly have known, as I gave that brief speech, that two decades later I would be writing a book on natural healing. But spreading the word about healing herbs is, after all, the most rewarding aspect of my work. I believe, as do many parents, that in addition to a repertoire of remedies that helps the body heal itself, the natural approach to wellness helps engage our young to be involved in their own health care, offering a level of understanding that will stay with them for their entire lives. They learn that taking care of their bodies preventatively is every bit as important as consulting a doctor when they are sick.

America's surge in interest for natural therapies to complement, and sometimes even replace, conventional medical treatment has been reflected in, as well as driven by, mainstream media. As a result, educational opportunities in the field of holistic health care have blossomed. Even our most respected medical schools are adding studies in natural therapies to their curricula. Think back to the 1970s, when massage was noted for its sexual connotations. Now it's a reimbursable medical expense under many health-care plans. I could not have imagined twenty years ago that *The New York Times* would have run a piece on "alternative medicine" and was delighted when they wrote about me and herbal remedies.

In the sixties and seventies, my father's losing battle with heart disease fostered my interest in alternative healing options. I have always believed in the adage "Seek and ye shall find," and that's precisely what I did. I was surprised to discover that natural healing therapies never went out of style in Europe and, in fact, that they have long been the primary modality of healing throughout much of the world. According to the World Health Organization, over 80% of the world uses herbs for healing!

My undergraduate work focused on speech pathology for children. Throughout the years, as an early childhood teacher, and mother of two sons, I continued to be actively involved with children. Positive feedback is great for building one's confidence, so after years of informally sharing my herbal remedies with friends and family, I followed my heart's desire and formalized my studies in herbology. Four years of study, in addition to field work and apprenticeships helped me to attain the level of Master Herbalist. I was privileged to be mentored in the work of the late Dr. John R. Christopher, one of the most respected authors and practitioners of natural health care in this country. Dr. Christopher lovingly shared his botanical formulas with the world, and, in the spirit of carrying on his tradition, I gladly share them with you in the chapters to follow.

I maintain a private practice for those people requiring a deeper level of assistance but continue to lecture nationwide, helping others to help themselves naturally. *Gentle Healing for Baby and Child* evolved in response to innumerable requests for a simple, straightforward guide for parents. Books on herbs are plentiful, but my research reveals that very few offer an easy, gentle approach for children. (Do consider using many of these therapies on yourselves. After all, what's good for little bodies also works on bigger bodies — it's just not always so in reverse.) As parents, we are especially cautious about how we treat our youngsters. A guideline for peace of mind is Andrea's Rule of Three:

- ✿ **Three days:** If you are dealing with an acute situation, expect it to be turned around within three days or seek medical help.
- ✿ **Three weeks:** For a gentle program of internal cleansing of organs, allow three weeks.
- ✿ **Three months:** To reverse a long-standing, chronic condition, create a three-month focus of healing therapies and lifestyle changes for your child.

All of the remedies presented here are perfectly safe, and are the result of years of experience with clients and, of course, my own sons, Chris and Brian. Best of all, incorporating these remedies into your children's lifestyles will teach them how important it is to be in charge of their own health, and the gift of health is, indeed, one of the greatest blessings of all.

As a Master Herbalist, I consider it an honor to be able to share over 25 years of experience with you, and to gently introduce you to the healing power of herbs. May this book be the cornerstone of your children's excellent health and wellness now, and for the rest of their lives.

Andrea Candee
South Salem, New York

2

A Brief History of Herbs

From the earliest of times, herbs have been hailed for their healing properties by civilizations in every corner of the globe. Today, approximately 25% of our doctor-prescribed medicines are based on one or more herbal ingredients, and many over-the-counter preparations contain botanicals as well.

There is strong evidence to support the fact that ancient cultures revered the curative powers of healing plants, and did so long before the development of the written word. The earliest proof may well be in the excavation of a 60,000-year-old burial site in Iraq that contained eight different medicinal plants.

Archaeologists and antiquities scholars have long known of the medicinal use of herbs from as early as 3,000 BC in Egypt, the Middle East, and China. Written evidence dates from around 1,500 BC in the form of Egyptian papyrus, which lists dozens of medicinal plants and their uses. Myrrh, castor oil, and garlic are all described, and their properties prized.

Written at about the same time, the Indian epic poems called Vedas contain substantial references to the herbal knowledge of that era. Around 700 BC, the Indian physician Charaka wrote a document called *Charaka Samhita*, which details the properties of over 300 herbal medicines, some of which are still in use today.

By the 2nd century AD, global trade routes had come into exis-
tence. It was the resultant cultural exchanges that allowed herbal
traditions to be circulated among civilizations in Europe, the
Middle East, and Asia. Cloves are the perfect example. Native to the
Philippines and South Pacific islands, cloves were imported to
China which, in turn, introduced these herbs to Egypt. By the 8th
century AD, their antiseptic and analgesic properties were known
throughout the European continent.

As the value of herbs grew, many writers and botanists tried to cat-
alog plants and to record their medicinal properties. Chief among
these works is the Chinese *Divine Husbandman's Classic (Shen'ong
Bencaojing)*, dating from the 1st century AD, and including 250
herbal medicines. Though sophisticated for its time, this text was
just a harbinger of the intricate Chinese herbal therapies that developed over the ages—and which, of course, form the basis of
Chinese medicine today.

Interestingly, a similar document was written at the same time by
a Greek physician called Dioscorides. His *De Materia Medica*, listing 600 herbs, is generally regarded as the first authoritative
European herbal text; it remained the pre-eminent book of its kind
until the 17th century, and was translated into various languages of
the world.

While the Middle Ages seemed like the Dark Ages in many
ways, this was much less the case when it came to herbs. Indeed,
historians have shown that Europeans of this time had a fairly
sophisticated knowledge of plant medicine. Excavations of an 11th
century monastic hospital in Scotland show that the monks were
using exotic herbs, including opium poppy and marijuana for their
pain-killing properties. (No, dear readers, I am not recommending
their use for your children!) Similarly, herbal practitioners in the
south Wales village of Myddfai, wrote texts that show a strong knowledge of the healing powers of plants.

Non-European cultures also recognized the medicinal properties
of herbs. The Ayurvedic tradition of India (whose Golden Age
occurred in the 7th century) was studied at universities, and medicinal herb gardens were popular throughout the country. At the same

time, the Mayas, Aztecs, and Incas all had extensive herbal traditions. Their use of sarsaparilla as a blood cleanser and skin healer indicates their understanding of herbs as medicinals.

Ironically, it was French mathematician René Descartes' notion of rationalism that squelched the herbal tradition in Europe in the early 17th century. While the Chinese and Indian cultures long accepted (and respected) the healing power of nature, the rationalist movement divided the world into distinct categories of body, mind, nature, and ideas. The orientation toward natural healing that had been long revered in Europe was suddenly seen as backward—despite the fact that French and English explorers in the New World continued to use herbal therapies and expanded their knowledge through their interactions with Indians indigenous to South America.

Nicholas Culpepper, a 17th-century English pharmacist, helped gain respect for botanical medicine during a time when British physicians were becoming contemptuous of natural medicine. His published herbals (essays on the uses of herbs) encouraged readers to use nature's pharmacy, herbs growing in their own backyards, to heal themselves. In so doing, they validated a long-standing tradition of English families. Today, many of Culpepper's recommendations are still in use.

The rationalist movement had taken such strong hold in Europe that, by 1858, the practice of medicine was banned by anyone who had not attended a conventional medical school. Fortunately, similar legislation was banned in France, Spain, and Italy; but in Britain, herbalists who continued to practice risked fines, imprisonment, or both. This ban actually led to the establishment of the National Institute of Medical Herbalists in 1864; it is to these steadfast souls that we owe a debt for having kept the herbal tradition alive.

Throughout the 20th century, herbal traditions continued quietly in Western Europe. However, they met their decline in the U.S. and Canada as breakthroughs in medical science were newly embraced. What helped turn the tide; why have so many North Americans rediscovered the holistic healing benefits of herbs and other natural therapies?

While advances in modern medicine have been brilliant, it is also true that more people today suffer from chronic illness and general disease than ever before. Medicine is terrific at treating acute ailments, but rather less successful at preventative health care and long-term wellness.

This is why the works of holistically oriented physicians like Drs. Andrew Weil and Dean Ornish have been widely embraced by the mainstream media and public. In response, Harvard and other top medical schools are now incorporating natural-healing techniques into their curricula, along with anatomy, pathology, and other conventional medical courses.

In the 1960s and '70s, the term "holistic medicine" indicated an emphasis on natural therapies for treating the entire body as a whole rather than just a body part. In the '80s, "complementary medicine" became the term of choice until the 1990s, when Dr. Weil coined the phrase "integrated medicine." We do not want to toss the baby with the bathwater, but instead take the best therapies from holistic and conventional medical practice from around the world and integrate them into a medical approach that can be flexible and life-enhancing. I am encouraged that the integrated approach will play a major role in the medical movement of the 21st century and in the future of our children's system of health care.

3

Dosing Guidelines

How to Dose Your Child

Since children at any given age can vary greatly in size and weight, I prefer to use weight rather than age as the most important factor in dosing children with herbs.

- ❀ To best determine the dose for your child, use an adult weight of 150 pounds as the baseline constant.
- ❀ Using the figure of 150 pounds as the common denominator, put your child's actual weight over it to determine a fraction of the standard adult dose. (Thus, if your boy or girl weighs 50 pounds and the standard baseline is 150, you will want to give ⅓ of the adult dose.)

$$\frac{50 \text{ pounds (child's weight)}}{150 \text{ pounds (baseline adult weight)}} = \text{⅓ dose}$$

The following general guidelines apply:

Child's Weight	Dosage
10 pounds	¹⁄₁₅ of adult dose
20 pounds	⅛ of adult dose

Child's Weight	*Dosage*
30 pounds	⅕ of adult dose
40 pounds	¼ of adult dose
50 pounds	⅓ of adult dose
60 pounds	⅖ of adult dose
70 pounds	½ of adult dose
80 pounds	½ of adult dose
90 pounds	⅗ of adult dose
100 pounds	⅔ of adult dose

Adult Doses

The amounts of ingestible forms of herbs can vary widely. The following is a general baseline from which to figure out your child's dose.

- Liquid extracts: 30 drops, 3–4 times a day
- Teas: 1 cup, 3–4 times a day
- Capsules: 2 capsules, 3–4 times a day
- Powdered herbs: ½ teaspoon, 3–4 times a day

Liquid extracts and powdered herbs may be diluted in 1–2 ounces breast milk, formula, or water.

Reduce Quantity, Not Frequency

When you calculate a child's dose according to weight, always reduce the *quantity* of the dose rather than its frequency.

- For example, an adult dose of 1 cup of medicinal tea to be administered 3–4 times a day translates into ⅓ cup, given 3–4 times daily for a 50-pound child.
- To make the math easier, it is often helpful to first convert

cups to ounces. For instance, an 8-ounce adult dose becomes 1 ounce for an infant of about 20 pounds.

How to Dose Eardrops

- ✿ The standard adult dose for eardrops is 3 to 4 drops in each ear.
- ✿ A toddler's dose would be 2 drops; an infant's, 1 drop in each ear.
- ✿ After treatment, to avoid an uncomfortable oily buildup in the ears, cleanse the ears by inserting a few drops of hydrogen peroxide.
- ✿ Here's another helpful hint: The easiest time to insert eardrops (especially for very young children) is when they are sleeping.

Cayenne Dosing

Although it is perceived as an irritating herb, cayenne in its raw state has demulcent, or soothing properties that result from its high mineral content. When cooked, cayenne changes chemically and becomes an irritant. To preserve its health-promoting properties, I recommend you add cayenne at the end of cooking rather than at the start of food preparation — if your family likes spicy foods!

The first question to be determined is: when is a child old enough for cayenne therapy? That's a decision best made with your child. Variables such as emotional maturity, compliance, self-confidence, and willingness to try new things enter into the decision. One child of eight may be more ready to try it than a child of twelve. Of course, the nature of the problem is also a factor. When an oral dose of cayenne is needed in an emergency situation, such as a severe nosebleed, treatment may have to prevail over readiness.

You can administer cayenne to your child in the form of a powder or liquid extract. I do not recommend cayenne capsules, as it is more beneficial if the child's esophageal fluids move the herb naturally down the digestive tract. The liquid extract of cayenne is available in health food stores, while the powdered cayenne can be found on the supermarket shelf. Perhaps there is already a supply of it in your pantry.

- The adult's therapeutic dose for cayenne is 15 to 20 drops (diluted in 2 ounces water or juice), 3 times a day.
- To build a tolerance for cayenne's hot sensation, begin dosing your child with a diluted drop or two, gradually building up to the full weight-appropriate dose.
- When given in powdered form, begin with ⅛ teaspoon (diluted in 1–2 ounces water or juice), 3 times a day. In an acute situation such as an asthma attack, cayenne may be given every 15–20 minutes for the first hour and once an hour thereafter until relief is attained.

The best way to give cayenne is as follows:

1. Put a favorite treat on the counter. (You'll see why later.)
2. Place the appropriate amount of cayenne in a shot glass. Add an ounce of water or juice.
3. In addition, have a full glass of water or juice on hand.
4. Have your child take the full contents of the shot glass in her mouth (at this point it won't burn) without swallowing it.
5. Have her add a mouthful of water/juice and swallow it all down together. Taking both the diluted cayenne solution and water/juice at the same time allows the cayenne to be further diluted as it goes down the throat, where it can burn.
6. Continue to give more water or juice until the discomfort subsides, which it does very quickly.
7. Here's where the treat comes into play. Doesn't the child in all of us need a reward for action that's "above and beyond"?

To relieve the burning sensation cayenne can leave in the throat, offer the eastern Indian accompaniment to hot, spicy foods: plain yogurt. The hot chemicals in cayenne dissolve in fat so be sure the yogurt is made from whole milk rather than the low-fat version. A swallow of whole milk, or, even tastier, a teaspoon of full-fat ice cream, can also cool the heat.

Garlic Dosing

FRESH CLOVES

Depending upon your child's age and preference, garlic can be used fresh—which is the best way to use it—or in perles, tablets, or oil, 3–4 times a day.

To give fresh garlic, you can:

- chop it and put on buttered toast (real garlic bread!)
- add to mashed potatoes
- put in a sandwich or salad
- cook with vegetables

Experiment to find out how much garlic your child will comfortably consume.

PERLES AND TABLETS

- One perle or tablet may be given to your child 3–4 times a day up to age 12.
- After 12 years of age, 2 tablets or perles are recommended.

GARLIC OIL

- Give 2–3 drops to an infant.
- 4 drops for a 4-year-old;
- 8 drops to an 8-year-old, until your child is old enough to swallow a perle or tablet.
- You can dilute the garlic oil in ¼–½ cup juice in a baby's bottle, or in a shot glass for toddlers and older children.

How to Administer Herbs to a Child

✿ Creativity is the key in getting your child to take herbs! The unfamiliar tastes can be masked or enhanced by the addition of a small amount of honey or fruit juice to a tea or liquid extract. (My sons liked apple and cranberry.)

✿ Using mini-cups and shot glasses is another way of making the dose seem less imposing.

When my son, Brian, was five, he had to take an extended course of a vile-tasting liquid extract—a concoction so unappealing that virtually nothing I tried could mask its taste. It took all of my ingenuity to figure out a way to get this into him 3 times a day without causing permanent trauma to us both! I took Brian to the grocery store to pick out a juice he'd never had before. Five Alive was new to the market, and he picked that one. But I insisted that the only way he could have his Five Alive was with his important herbal medicine. The technique, I must say, worked like a charm. I never brought that juice into the house after the therapy was over, and when he was older and tried some on his own, he was surprised it didn't taste at all as he had remembered!

✿ Teas that you use for ongoing therapy, such as for blood/liver cleansing or digestive support, can be steeped a little stronger and frozen into ice pops (always a favorite with Chris). Note, however, that respiratory issues respond best to warm infusions of tea.

✿ If your child cannot swallow a capsule, you may mix its powdered contents with a little applesauce.

✿ For the nursing child, the benefits of herbal therapy may be had via mother's milk. Mother needs to drink more frequent doses of an herbal infusion or decoction so that the healing properties pass into her bloodstream and thus into her milk—and into the child's system as well.

✿ Spearmint is a marvelous way to mask the flavor of a tea. Its refreshing taste and aroma can transform the experience into a most pleasant one.

✿ To administer tea or another liquid to your infant, I suggest using an eyedropper. Fill it first with the correct dose of the herb, then draw up some water or juice. Pull your baby's cheek out and deposit the dose in the mouth.

4

Herbs to the Rescue!

Back in the days when I was just a budding herbalist—please forgive the pun—I considered every one of my active sons' scrapes and bruises the chance to use my newfound knowledge. When they fell off their bikes or out of a tree, Chris and Brian went from offspring to clients in a moment's time!

Most parents prefer to introduce herbal healing (indeed, "alternative" therapies of any kind) to their children gingerly. These suggestions for the rough and tumble mishaps of youth are a good place to start because they are among the easiest to use. In fact, many of these remedies are much less invasive and better liked by kids than the standard first aid practices you may currently be using.

SPLINTERS

Whether it's a splinter, sliver of glass, remaining tick part, or any other unwanted foreign object, the customary plan of attack is to go in after it with a sterilized needle. Rather than expecting your child to withstand this uncomfortable exploration or worse, leaving it alone in peril of becoming painfully red, swollen and infected, call forth the banana as hero of the day. A ripened banana peel is rich in digestive enzymes. It is the drawing action of the enzymes that will pull the foreign matter to the surface of the skin.

I guarantee this is a remedy your child will broadcast to the neighborhood, and that it will catch on like wildfire. It certainly did in my neck of the woods!

The Banana Trick

- ✿ Cut a piece of ripened banana peel to cover the affected area.
- ✿ Apply the pulp side of the banana peel against the skin
- ✿ Hold the banana peel in place with a piece of surgical tape. (See Appendix A for a description of the type of surgical tape I have found to work best.)
- ✿ Leave on overnight. In the morning, the banana will have drawn the foreign matter to the surface, ready for easy removal—or, better still, may show in the peel when you remove it from the skin. More deeply embedded splinters may require one or two more nights of this treatment, in which case you should use a fresh section of peel each time.

The Sticky Tape Trick

Oftentimes a splinter can be easily removed with a pair of tweezers because it has not become deeply embedded but wouldn't it be more fun (and less intimidating) to use sticky tape instead!

- ✿ Cut a piece of tape to cover the splinter and surrounding area.
- ✿ Gently press down on the tape so that it adheres to the splinter.
- ✿ Slowly pull the tape back in the direction in which the splinter should be removed.
- ✿ With the splinter stuck to the tape you can affix it to a piece of paper and have your child incorporate it into a fun drawing.

FROM CUTS AND SCRAPES TO BLEEDING WOUNDS

Day-to-day skinned knees and scraped elbows can easily be treated with one of the remedies described in this section. More serious, bleeding wounds can also be handled with the herbal information provided.

When do you decide that you need professional help in handling your child's injury? While the remedies described here have proved their mettle in emergency situations, it's really a subjective call. You'll know within the first few minutes what is beyond your comfort zone. No matter how brave you are, seek help if:

- ✿ The injury has caused a wide or jagged split in the skin.
- ✿ The wound is too deep to cleanse without an anesthetic.
- ✿ The bleeding persists.
- ✿ Your child is vomiting, dizzy, fainting, or exhibiting any uncontrollable response.

The Disappearing Blood Trick

To prevent your child the trauma of seeing his or her own blood, here's a trick I used with my own boys: Wash the area with a red or dark-colored washcloth. The event seems less frightening, and allows for a more cooperative child who is engaged in his or her own healing process.

Nature's Soothers

In most cases, superficial injuries require no more attention than a cleansing and a kiss. Sometimes a little more attention is needed both for the comforting of spirits (your child's and yours) and the soothing of the injury. The following herbal remedies, available at any health food store, gently relieve sore, inflamed skin with their anti-inflammatory properties as well as accelerate its healing.

Mullein flower oil
St. John's Wort oil
Aloe gel
Castor oil
Ointment infused with comfrey, calendula, and/or burdock root

- ❀ After cleansing with soap and water or an herbal wash (see below), completely cover the injured skin and its surrounding area with one of the above herbal preparations.
- ❀ Reapply treatment 2–3 times a day.
- ❀ While exposure to air aids the healing process, depending upon the location of the injury, you may need to keep the area bandaged for a couple of days to protect it from being irritated by clothing. Also, a bandage will help keep the preparation concentrated on the injured skin.
- ❀ The herbal applications may be continued throughout the healing process to prevent the uncomfortable feeling that comes with scabbing.
- ❀ The reassuring thing about using these preparations is that you can never overdo them. You can stop using them when your child no longer feels a need for them.

Honey: Nature's Skin Healer

It may surprise you to find honey included in this section on healing cuts. Honey has been used worldwide in modern medical arenas. For example, in World War I, German physicians mixed honey with cod liver oil to treat battlefield wounds. In third world countries, where antibiotics may be scarce, honey is routinely applied to cuts and sores as a disinfectant.

Referenced in their medical text, the Smith Papyrus (2600–2200 BC), the ancient Egyptians used honey as did Hippocrates, the Greek physician, for skin ailments, wounds, cuts, and burns.

Used universally for thousands of years as an ingredient in salves, honey has been thoroughly studied for its anti-microbial properties.

The Lancet, the British medical journal, reported that honey produces natural hydrogen peroxide at the site of a wound, which helps to accelerate healing and protect against infection.

Honey may be safely used topically for infants, children, and adults. It should not be given internally to babies under the age of one year because their digestive systems may not have developed enough to handle the deadly botulism bacteria that sometimes contaminates honey. The Center for Disease Control reports that cases of infant botulism are rare, but not worth the risk.

The honey will keep the skin supple so that the forming scab doesn't feel tight, itchy, and uncomfortable. I can't think of a sweeter way to soothe your sweetie's scraped knee.

- ❀ After cleansing the area with soap and water or an herbal wash (see below), coat the injured skin and its surrounding area with enough honey to form a thick, protective layer.
- ❀ Apply the "honey bandage" twice a day.
- ❀ Cover with gauze and surgical tape for a day or two to keep the area protected and the honey in place. The covering will also keep the honey treatment from being a messy one.
- ❀ You may continue applying a thin coating of honey after the skin has scabbed over, for as long as is needed, to keep the area feeling comfortable.
- ❀ If your jar of honey has become crystallized, restore it to its liquid state by warming the jar in hot water until the crystals dissolve.

Antiseptic Washes

While the cleansing of the injury is absolutely essential to prevent infection, it can be a scary, painful event for a child. Distraction can work wonders: sing, whistle, exchange silly jokes!

To cleanse wounds, you can use an infusion of herbs as an antiseptic wash. Consider sage, chamomile, or calendula for anti-inflammatory and anti-microbial properties.

- ❀ Cover 3 teaspoons of the herb (or any combination of the herbs) with a cup of boiled water and allow to steep for 5 minutes while you are comforting your child.

   ❀ Use an ice cube to cool the solution to a temperature comfortable to the skin.

   ❀ Pour it gently and continuously over the affected area for deep and effective cleansing or pour into a spray bottle and spray on for an even gentler approach.

   ❀ The herbal-tea/antiseptic wash may be stored in the refrigerator for three days.

The Brown Paper Bag Trick

An old family method to stop the bleeding of minor cuts is to use a brown paper bag as a compression bandage. Brown paper bags seemed always to be around, used for garbage, groceries, and school lunches. In the same way men often stop their shaving cuts from bleeding with a bit of tissue, a piece of brown paper bag can quickly be torn off to be used as a pressure bandage, applying firmly to the cut. I can remember several incidences arising with my boys, at home in the kitchen, in the supermarket, even in the car after going grocery shopping, where a quick tear from the bag became a fast first aid tool.

   ❀ Make a "bandage" from brown paper torn from a grocery bag and tape or firmly hold on the cut.

   ❀ Leave in place until the bleeding stops.

Cayenne Pepper to the Rescue

High in Vitamin K, the clotting properties of the cayenne pepper will stop a child's bleeding within 10 seconds—a dramatic remedy, to say the least. Interestingly, cayenne's high mineral content lends to it the classification of a demulcent (a soothing herb); thus, despite its fiery reputation, it does not burn the skin, even when placed on a sensitive wound.

- ✿ Spoon a thick layer of powdered cayenne onto the affected area.
- ✿ Cover with a bandage; leave on overnight. The bleeding will stop within 10 seconds.

What's more, cayenne's antimicrobial and astringent properties will help cleanse and close the cut. You do not have to wash the cayenne out of the cut as it is healing, because the cayenne comes off with the removal of the bandage.

Note: Head wounds are characterized by their ability to bleed excessively. Don't be alarmed. The cayenne pepper remedy even stopped the profuse bleeding from an injury to my son's head. After the bleeding has stopped, check your child for signs of concussion (dizziness, blurred vision, headache, weakness, nausea, vomiting) and have a medical checkup to be sure there is no undetected internal hemorrhaging.

Rescue Remedy

I don't have to tell you that any deep wound is as emotionally invasive as the wound itself. So I use the following natural nerve-calmer to help restore equilibrium to a child's state of mind.

- ✿ Place 4 drops Rescue Remedy (see Bach Flower Essences in Appendix I) in ½ glass water and allow the child to sip the mixture during and after the treatment.
- ✿ Once the bleeding has stopped (or, in the case of a cayenne poultice, the next day, after the bandage has been removed), you can apply one of the herbal preparations described above to speed healing.

Comfrey

Given its cell proliferant properties, I find that fresh or powdered comfrey is the best natural skin healer there is. It encourages the regrowth of skin cells and thus is ideal for packing into a deep wound.

❀ If using fresh comfrey leaves, mascerate them in a blender. If using dried leaf or root, mix 1 tablespoon of the powdered herb with just enough water to make a paste.

❀ Apply a thick layer of the fresh pulp or powdered herb paste to the affected area and cover with a bandage.

❀ The wound will absorb the comfrey. For the first few days, check it 3 times a day, and add more comfrey, as needed. Do not remove the old plant material; simply add more to what is already there.

❀ After the wound has closed, any of the herbal preparations mentioned above may be applied to promote further healing and relieve discomfort.

Garlic

During World War II, the British used the well-documented, powerful anti-microbial properties of garlic to treat wounds, thereby preventing septic poisoning in their soldiers. You can do the same at home for wounds that contain debris or are difficult to cleanse. This garlic poultice can be used after cleansing the site to prevent infection or be called upon to heal an existing infection.

The signs to look for when skin is infected are:

Reddened, inflamed skin
Painful swelling
Fluid oozing from the wound
A foul smell coming from the injured site

Garlic Poultice

❀ Remove two cloves from a bulb of garlic. Peel and finely mince.

❀ Place the garlic in the center of a 2" square of cheesecloth, folding over the edges to make a packet.

❀ Cover the infected area with the cheesecloth packet.

❀ Bind in place with roller gauze and surgical tape.

☙ Apply a fresh poultice twice a day until the skin looks like it is healing healthfully.

BURNS

As safe as we try to make our homes for our children, they're loaded with danger. Household chemicals, cooking appliances, electrical equipment and outlets are part of their everyday environment. Sometimes little hands reach for pots, hot plates, or wires even before we have a chance to warn them. Whatever the severity of the burn, immediate action must be taken.

When to Seek Emergency Help

Burns that appear more than reddened or mildly blistered should be immediately seen by your doctor or emergency room personnel. If the skin is charred or severely blistered, do not bathe it in water. If clothing or anything else is attached to the skin, leave it alone. Simply cover the area with a clean cotton cloth and allow the area to be professionally treated.

You can give your child Rescue Remedy (see Bach Flower Essences in Appendix I) to sip for shock and trauma while seeking emergency help—and you might like to sip some, too!

Natural Remedies for Burns

☙ Burns that seem manageable at home should be immediately bathed in cold water or cooled with cold water compresses for several minutes (use a soft cotton cloth such as a diaper, cotton napkin, or old sheet or pillowcase torn into strips). This helps reduce the pain and inflammation, and prevents the burn from penetrating deeper into the skin.

☙ Completely cover the burned area with the remedy you choose and cover with a bandage.

☙ If the area is too sensitive to be touched with the herbal preparation, use it to saturate a piece of gauze large enough to cover the burn and its surrounding tissue.

  ❀ Reapply 2–3 times a day.

  ❀ The herbal preparations can be used for as long as you feel necessary. Prolonged use will promote healing and after a day or two the bandage will probably no longer be needed.

  ❀ **Vitamin E.** Puncture a vitamin E capsule with a straight pin, and spread a thick layer of the oil on the burned skin. I always keep a bottle of vitamin E oil in my kitchen.

  ❀ **Lavender oil.** This is one of the only essential oils that can be applied directly to the skin without dilution.

  ❀ **St. John's Wort Oil.** Apply undiluted to the burn.

  ❀ **Comfrey ointment.** Apply directly on the burn.

Dr. Christopher's Burn Ointment

This is one of Dr. Christopher's most famous and well-used treatments for burns. The herbal ingredients are anti-inflammatory and anti-microbial. They soothe tissue and encourage growth of new skin. It can be used for severely reddened and blistered burns (if you feel comfortable handling them at home), or can be used a few days after medical treatment, with your doctor's approval.

  ❀ Mix together 1 tablespoon each powdered comfrey root, honey, wheat germ oil.

If you prefer, as a benefit of honey's preservative properties, a larger quantity of the herbal mixture can be prepared and stored for a few days at room temperature.

  ❀ Cover the burned area and its surrounding tissue with a thick coating of the herbal mixture.

  ❀ Cover with a bandage. Check dressing twice a day. The ointment will be absorbed by the body. Add more ointment without removing old material.

  ❀ When the body is no longer absorbing the mixture as quickly, replenish once a day until the site is completely renewed with freshly grown skin.

❀ To reduce the possibility of scarring, continue applying the wheat germ oil or apply castor oil until the skin has been totally restored.

Baby Bear's Burn Remedy

Raw, natural honey (purchased in a health food store) is a sweet, sticky way to ease the pain of a mild burn. Its antimicrobial and hydrating properties work to keep the area free of infection and well moisturized. Scientific study of honey indicates that its trace amounts of vitamins, minerals, antioxidants, and amino acids help make it an effective treatment for burns, scrapes, and minor sore throats.

❀ Gently apply a thick coating to take the hurt away in just seconds!

❀ Cover with gauze to keep the honey from messing clothing.

❀ Apply twice a day until the area is no longer sensitive.

Amazing Aloe Cure

While preparing dinner, I accidentally scalded myself with boiling water. Even after bathing the area in cold water for several minutes, the resulting burn proved to be too much for my old standby, vitamin E. When the vitamin E oil sizzled as it was applied to the burn, I knew a more powerful botanical therapy was required. My lovely aloe plant—something no household should be without— was standing ready to be pressed into service.

Aloe has the unique ability to help skin renew itself by stimulating cellular metabolism, thereby promoting oxygen exchange and increasing the absorption of nutrients. Aloe contains the antioxidant vitamins A and C; the minerals copper, selenium, and magnesium; and zinc, a powerful virus fighter.

✿ Rather than cutting from the tip or half way down the stalk, cut it at its base. Slit the stalk horizontally, exposing the gelatinous interior.

✿ Using the thickest, juiciest section for the burn, cut a piece large enough to completely cover the burn and its surrounding tissue. Place the entire piece on the area (gel and peel, gel side toward the burn).

✿ Cover the aloe with roller gauze and surgical tape to keep it firmly in place. (See *Note,* below.)

✿ Leave the dressing on overnight or, if the burn occurred early in the day, cut a fresh piece of aloe to make a new dressing and leave on overnight.

✿ The remaining stalk of aloe may be wrapped in plastic wrap and refrigerated overnight. In the morning, cut a new piece of the refrigerated aloe to make a fresh dressing.

✿ Repeat applications twice a day until area is healed.

Note: In the situation I described above, I made one mistake: I failed to bind the aloe securely. In the morning, the area covered by the gel alone was still hot, reddened, and blistered. The area covered by the gel and peel, however, was totally healed—not even a hint of redness remained! This taught me how important it is to cover a burn with both the gel and peel of the aloe plant.

SUNBURN

Parents know to limit the amount of time children spend in the sun and to cover them with protective lotion. That having been said, even the most careful parents can let their families get overexposed.

If sunburn does occur, the pain and inflammation can be relieved by any of the formulations presented above for burns or try one of these time-tested sunburn soothers.

Apple Cider Vinegar Bath

For large sunburned areas, an apple cider vinegar bath works wonders. Use a brand from the health food store that has been wood-
aged, rather than one from the supermarket that may have been
chemically aged. Apple cider vinegar helps to balance the skin's pH
factor, its acid/alkaline balance. As with all parts of the body, when
there is chemical balance, healing is supported.

- ❀ Add two cups apple cider vinegar to a bathtub of warm water.
- ❀ Let your child soak for 15 minutes. The skin will be calmed
  and soothed, and much of the pain will be immediately
  relieved.
- ❀ After the bath, you can use one of the burn remedies described
  above to promote further healing.

Yogurt Skin Healer

Though it may not have all of us living to 120 (remember those
Russian-peasant ads of several years back?), yogurt is a natural
healer. It is the antidote for the burn of hot, spicy food in Indian
cooking by reestablishing acid/alkaline balance and works the same
way for sunburned skin. For sunburn, I use compresses of natural
yogurt to help cool and hydrate the skin.

- ❀ Wrap whole-milk, plain yogurt in several layers of cheesecloth
  and compress the burn.
- ❀ Replace with fresh compresses as the yogurt warms on the
  skin. Repeat compresses until the skin is cooled and soothed.
- ❀ Yogurt can be spread over the entire body—turning an upsetting, painful sunburn into a fun spa treatment that girls, especially, will love. (And boys, too: My son Brian has always
  enjoyed our herbal "spa treatments.") Leave the yogurt on for
  10–15 minutes, then rinse off in a cool shower.

Baking Soda Sunburn Soother

No apple cider vinegar or plain yogurt in the house? Then check the deepest recess of your refrigerator for that box of baking soda you stashed there eons ago (hopefully, not too many eons—to effectively deodorize your fridge, baking soda should be changed about every 3 months). Like apple cider vinegar and yogurt, baking soda helps to balance pH, the skin's acid/alkaline balance.

❀ Add ¼ cup baking soda to a warm bath for an effective sunburn-healing soak.

❀ Have your child soak for 15 minutes.

Aloe Vera Plant

I consider an aloe vera plant an absolute necessity for healing burns, cuts, and sunburns. It requires a sunny window or indirect bright light and very little care (I water mine only twice a month). On page 27 I explain how to use the fresh plant. There are aloe products available in the health food store that might say 99% pure aloe. Indeed, the aloe that is in the product may be 99% pure but what part of the total product is actually aloe vera we do not know. To get the most out of this potent healer, I recommend using it fresh.

Soupy, Goopy Burn Gel

Whisk together and apply to affected areas, reapplying as often as needed:

½ cup gel scraped from the inside of the spear of the aloe vera plant
1 teaspoon vitamin E oil or 1 teaspoon wheat germ oil
  (or the equivalent from punctured capsules)
10 drops essential oil of lavender

❀ Taking the best of my favorite sunburn remedies, this poultice soothes, calms, and protects tender, sunburned skin.

❀ It can be gently patted onto large areas (best to wear an old T-shirt and shorts to prevent soiling good clothing).

❀ If using on just a forearm, for example, the area can be covered with roller gauze. Use your judgment as to what would be the most comfortable.

❀ If another application is required the following day, make up a fresh batch.

BROKEN BONES

It goes without saying that a broken bone requires immediate medical attention. If you suspect your child has a broken bone, don't guess; take your child to the nearest emergency room at once.

Certainly, resetting and casting the bone is of prime importance. But here we have excellent examples of how natural healing can complement modern medicine beautifully.

Calming the Nerves

While waiting or en route, I advise giving your child my favorite nerve-calmer, Rescue Remedy (see Bach Flower Essences in Appendix I).

❀ Place 4 drops Rescue Remedy in ½ cup water.

❀ Have your child sip the mixture immediately after the injury and at 15 minute intervals, until calm.

❀ You can give him the Rescue Remedy several times a day for the next few days following the accident.

❀ Don't forget to mix up a solution of Rescue Remedy for yourself!

Dr. Christopher's BF&C (Bone, Flesh, & Cartilage)

To promote the healing of broken bones and surrounding tissue, I recommend giving your child one dose of BF&C three times a day. One dose equals:

Ages 1–3 years	¼ of the capsule's powdered contents, mixed into food or liquid
Ages 4–5	½ of the capsule's powdered contents, mixed into food or liquid
Ages 6–12	1 capsule
Ages 12 and over	2 capsules

Every parent to whom I have recommended this formula has found that their child's bones healed more quickly than the doctor's original expectations.

Why does Dr. Christopher's BF& C work so well? Let's look at its ingredients and how they work in this formula: (See Appendix G for a note on comfrey.)

Herb	*Function*
Oak bark	Astringent, anti-inflammatory
Mullein leaf	Astringent, calms nerves
Black walnut leaf	Antiseptic, antimicrobial
Marshmallow root	Soothing, anti-inflammatory
Comfrey root	Cell proliferant, anti-inflammatory
Wormwood	Nerve tonic
Lobelia	Antispasmodic, nerve nourisher, strengthens muscular action of vessel walls
Skullcap	Nerve tonic, antispasmodic
Gravel root	Nerve tonic

Quantum Herbal Products (800–348–0398) makes an excellent enhanced liquid version of this formula.

Healing Visualizations

I often encourage my clients to use healing visualizations. Today, even conventionally trained physicians are embracing the healing power of thought. I highly recommend Dr. Gerald Epstein's books, *Healing Visualizations: Creating Health Through Imagery* (Bantam, 1989) and *Healing Into Immortality* (Bantam, 1994 and Acmi, 1996). A selection of visualization techniques can also be found on p. 234.

Bone-Loving Tea

A few last words on broken bones. In many cultures, a cup of tea is a good "cure" for whatever ails you. In the case of a broken bone, the calming and anti-inflammatory properties of chamomile can assist recovery, as does the high silica content of oatstraw and horsetail. (Silica is a material that assists the body in absorbing calcium from supplements and food, and calcium, as you know, is an important mineral for the healing of bone tissue.)

- ⚘ Combine 1 teaspoon each dried chamomile flowers, oatstraw, and horsetail leaves.
- ⚘ Cover with 1 cup boiled water and steep for 30 minutes.
- ⚘ Strain and serve in 2–4 oz. doses up to age 5; 4–6 oz. doses up to age 12; 8 oz. doses age 12 and over.
- ⚘ Give this concentrated form of Bone-Loving Tea to your child 3 times a day for 3 months to promote a stronger healing of the broken bone and its surrounding tissue.
- ⚘ For variety's sake, you can make the flavor of this tea more interesting by adding some of your child's favorite fruit juice.

BRUISES, SPRAINS, STRAINS, SPORTS INJURIES

When you have two children as athletically inclined as I do, they provide great opportunities for the "lowly" onion to strut its healing stuff. Onion, high in sulfur compounds, is known for its ability to open channels, encouraging the thinning and flowing of fluids (as in tear ducts, something all cooks know about!), but it does far more than that. By virtue of its ability to discourage aggregation of blood cells, it can actually reduce the swelling associated with forceful contact of all kinds—sports injuries, falls, bumps, etc. Applying ice will reduce swelling, but the onion does far more: it also minimizes pain and promotes healing by moving stagnant cellular material which was called forth to protect the body at the moment of impact. As a result, you can expect less bruising.

When one of my sons was injured on the playing field, I restrained myself from running out to my "baby" to wrap him in something strange. (Remember, even 10 years ago, any kind of natural remedy was considered circumspect and odd by most—no *Newsweek* cover stories back then.) So I allowed the coach to apply ice and a rah-rah pat on the back; but as soon as we got home, I whipped out my trusty onion.

Smelly Yellow Onion Debruiser and Sprain Remedy

- ✿ Affix a ¼" slice of yellow onion to the bruise using surgical tape, covering with plastic wrap, if desired.
- ✿ Leave on for several hours or overnight. You'll find it amazing how soon the onion reduces the pain, inflammation, and residue black and blue of the injury.

This also works well for sprained fingers.

- ✿ Cut a piece of onion to comfortably fit and apply to injury.
- ✿ Cover with plastic wrap; tape to secure it.
- ✿ Leave on overnight.

One caveat, however: never apply onion directly to broken skin. If you've ever done so (even inadvertently, in the kitchen), you know that this can hurt far more than the injury itself.

Castor Oil

The oil of the castor bean helps speed up lymphatic flow and reduces inflammation, helping to reduce black-and-blue pain and discoloration.

- ❀ Apply a thin layer of castor oil to the bruise twice a day.
- ❀ For a large area (an arm, leg, or thigh) where the skin has been broken, use one of the remedies discussed above for cuts and scrapes, then cover with a castor oil pack. Even if the skin has not been broken, you can use this pack to help restore good circulation to the area. (See Appendix A for a description of the benefits and application of a castor oil pack.)

Castor oil packs may be used to:

Soothe a tummyache
Relieve strained or sprained muscles
Reduce internal pain while waiting for appropriate plan of action
    to take effect
Calm an agitated nervous system
Promote restful sleep

St. John's Wort Bruiseaway

The anti-inflammatory and nerve-toning properties of St. John's Wort reduce inflammation and sensitivity at injured nerve endings (as in a pinched finger or stubbed toe).

- ❀ Apply a thin coating of the oil of St. John's Wort to the affected area 3–4 times a day.
- ❀ If desired, moisten gauze with the oil and affix to the injured area with surgical tape.

Arnica Oil

Arnica is well known throughout Europe for its analgesic and anti-inflammatory properties. I find it works best when used immediately after a bruise, sprain, or strain. Apply as described above for *St. John's Wort Bruiseaway*.

Dr. Christopher's BF&C Ointment (Bone, Flesh, & Cartilage)

The herbs in this wonderful ointment (see section on broken bones for a full list of its ingredients and healing properties) soothe the injury and relieve discomfort. Moreover, it's something your child can easily reapply several times a day, if desired, thereby taking an active part in the healing process, which fosters emotional as well as physical comfort.

That said, we all know that your kisses to the bruised area are just as essential at any age (okay, at least until graduate school) as the primary healing agent!

Comfrey Poultice

Allantoin, one of comfrey's outstanding chemical ingredients, reduces inflammation. Rosmarinic acid, another constituent of this wonderful healing herb, reduces swelling. This dynamic duo brings powerful relief to the discomforts of bruises, sprains, and strains.

- ✿ If using fresh comfrey leaves, mascerate in blender with enough water to cover.
- ✿ Place as much of the mixture as you can on the affected area.
- ✿ Cover with gauze and surgical tape. Leave in place overnight.
- ✿ If the poultice is still required in the morning, replace with a fresh mixture.
- ✿ If using dried, powdered comfrey, mix up enough of the powder with water to make a paste that fully covers the affected area. Proceed as above.

❀ The comfrey poultice may be reapplied 2–3 times a day for as many days as is needed to reduce pain and swelling.

Inflammation and Pain

Discomforts associated with injuries may require herbs with anti-inflammatory, antiseptic, nervine, and/or analgesic properties. Choose from the list below, based upon your child's needs. Any and all of the following herbs can be combined.

Please do not feel intimidated by the amount of choices provided. They give you the opportunity to be flexible and creative while bringing emotional and physical relief to your child.

See the example given at the end of this section to see how easily a healing protocol can be developed.

Analgesic Herbs (to reduce pain)

White willow bark, meadowsweet, cat's claw

❀ Give in the form of a tea, liquid extract, or capsule 3 times a day. See dosing schedule in Chapter 3 for amounts.

Arnica gel, ointment, or oil

❀ Thickly coat the surface of the injury and its surrounding tissue 3 times a day.

Homeopathic arnica

❀ Give homeopathic arnica every few hours (sold in health food stores and many pharmacies), allowing the sweet-tasting pellet to dissolve under the tongue. When using homeopathic preparations (herbs that are in extremely dilute form), nothing can be had to eat or drink 20 minutes before and after the dose is given; otherwise, it will be rendered ineffective.

❇ These delicate remedies can be antidoted by the oils in your skin so instead of handling them, tap the dose into the cap provided and drop the pellet into your child's mouth.

❇ Give one pellet to children under 10 and two pellets to children over 10 years of age.

Anti-Inflammatory Herbs (to reduce reddened and/or swollen areas, irritation)

White willow bark, meadowsweet, cat's claw

❇ Give in the form of a tea, liquid extract, or capsule three times a day. See dosing schedule in Chapter 3 for amounts.

Arnica gel, ointment, or oil, aloe gel, St. John's Wort oil, calendula ointment or oil

❇ Thickly coat the surface of the injury and its surrounding tissue 3 times a day.

Chamomile, witch hazel leaf and bark, comfrey leaf and root

❇ Steep 2 teaspoons herb (or combination of herbs) in one cup boiled water for 30 minutes.
❇ Let cool until comfortable to the touch or speed up the cooling process with an ice cube; strain.
❇ Dip cloth into tea, wring out so it's not drippy, and compress (gently apply to) area 3–4 times a day.

Bromelain is an enzyme found in the stem (also in the fruit, but commercially prepared from the stem) of the pineapple plant.

❇ Its anti-inflammatory properties can help your child to more quickly and comfortably recover from an injury, fall, and even surgery, by reducing pain, tenderness, and swelling.
❇ The adult dose in such circumstances is 1000 mg given three

times a day. Consult dosing guidelines in Chapter 3 to determine the appropriate dosage for your child.

✿ Be sure to give bromelain at least half an hour away from food
so that it functions as an anti-inflammatory rather than a digestive enzyme.

Antiseptic Herbs (to cleanse, prevent infection)

Sage, calendula, thyme

✿ Cover 6 teaspoons of the herb (or any combination of the
herbs) with 2 cups boiled water and allow to steep for 3–5 minutes while you are comforting your child.
✿ Use an ice cube to cool the solution to a temperature comfortable to the skin.
✿ Pour it gently and continuously over the affected area for deep
and effective cleansing or pour into a spray bottle and spray on
for an even gentler approach.
✿ Do not recycle the liquid: once it has been poured over the
injured area do not reuse.

Tea tree, thyme

✿ Mix 3 drops essential oil in one-half cup water.
✿ Pour it gently and continuously over the affected area for deep
and effective cleansing or pour into a spray bottle and spray on
for an even gentler approach.
✿ Do not recycle the liquid: once it has been poured over the
injured area do not reuse.

Nervine Herbs (to relax the emotions and body)

Passionflower, hops, valerian, lemon balm, chamomile, wild oats,
catnip, skullcap

✿ Give in the form of a tea, liquid extract, or capsule as needed.

See dosing schedule in Chapter 3 for amounts.

Lavender, lemon balm, neroli (orange blossom)

⚘ Add 3–5 drops essential oil to bath water.
⚘ Have your child breathe deeply to inhale the aromatic benefits of the herb.
⚘ Encourage quiet play while bathing.

Lavender, lemon balm, orange blossom, Roman chamomile

⚘ Add 3 drops essential oil to a tablespoon of almond oil.
⚘ Give your child a gentle, relaxing body massage.

Lavender, lemon balm

⚘ A few drops of essential oil can be placed on a pillowcase or on the bulb of a night-light.

Here's an example of how the above herbs were put into action:
Five-year-old Nicholas was injured in a playground fall. He suffered a painful abrasion on his thigh. Making her choices from the herbs outlined above, his mother:

⚘ Cleansed the area with a sage tea wash.
⚘ Applied aloe gel topically.
⚘ Gave him 10 drops (diluted in juice) of a pain-relieving, calming "cocktail" every few hours comprised of equal parts white willow bark and passionflower.
⚘ Gave Nicholas one pellet homeopathic arnica every few hours.

MUSCLE STRESS AND SPASMS

Often associated with injury or poor vertebral alignment, muscle stress and spasms are the result of blocked circulation in the affected area. For this reason, herbs that stimulate circulation are helpful. Look for ointments or oils that contain any of the following herbs:

Cayenne, ginger, peppermint, eucalyptus, St. John's Wort, arnica, lavender, castor oil

- ❀ Thickly coat the surface of the injury and its surrounding tissue 3 times a day.
- ❀ If desired, cover the area with a bandage.

Nervines, herbs that help calm the body, also help relax muscles: Valerian, passionflower, skullcap, hops, lemon balm

- ❀ Give in the form of a tea, liquid extract, or capsule as needed. See dosing schedule in Chapter 3 for amounts.

Nutritional deficiencies may also be a cause of muscular discomforts. High sugar intake affects the body's mineral balance which could result in muscle stress and/or spasms.

- ❀ The cell salt Mag. Phos. (see page 238 for a description of Cell Salts) helps to reestablish mineral balance.
- ❀ Give two pellets every 15 minutes until relief is attained (up to two hours).
- ❀ Allow the sweet-tasting pellets to dissolve under the tongue.
- ❀ When using homeopathic preparations (herbs that are in extremely dilute form), nothing can be had to eat or drink 20 minutes before and after the dose is given; otherwise, it will be rendered ineffective.
- ❀ Do not handle the pellets as the oils in your skin may render them ineffective. Instead, tap the dose into the bottle's cap and then tap into your child's mouth.

RESTLESS LEG SYNDROME

This can often be a result of a calcium/magnesium imbalance. Sugar intake must be addressed and reduced in the diet, as sugar can throw off the delicate balance of minerals in the body.

I have found the cell salt Mag. Phos. to be especially helpful in calming a jumpy leg. See directions above.

CHIROPRACTIC/OSTEOPATHY

An adjustment of the spine may provide quick relief, especially after a fall or accident. A chiropractor can correct subluxations of the spine (vertebral bones that may have slipped out of place).

An osteopath or practitioner of cranial-sacral technique adjusts the bones in the head as well as the spine. Their approaches are quite different, and each should be explored to determine which therapy is right for your child.

STIFF NECK

Neck problems affect young and old alike. Causes range from stress and injury (a tumble on the playing field, a car accident, etc.) to having slept wrong the night before. Nervine and anti-inflammatory herbs described above may help as well as a visit to a chiropractor or osteopath.

If your child's stress seems to consistently settle in the neck and shoulder area, try to address the cause of the stress. (See the section on Mindful Living in Chapter 11.) You can also teach this adaptation of a wonderful exercise devised by Edgar Cayce, a 20th-century medical intuitive. You might want to do this along with your child to relieve some of your own neck tension—I certainly did!

The Tension-Taming Neck Game

Make this a fun exercise by stating: "I can see . . ." after each stretch, showing your child how much flexibility is progressively gained as indicated by how much more they can see.

Repeat each step 3 times before moving on to the next one. Breathe in deeply during the first part of each step, and exhale during the return to starting position.

1. Looking straight ahead, gently tilt the head to look up at the ceiling; return to starting position.
2. Looking straight ahead, gently lower chin to chest; return to starting position.
3. Looking straight ahead, gently turn head to look over right shoulder; return to starting position.
4. Looking straight ahead, gently turn head to look over left shoulder; return to starting position.
5. With chin to chest, slowly rotate chin to right shoulder, point it up to the ceiling, over to left shoulder, and back down to chest.
6. With chin to chest, reverse above rotation by rotating chin to left shoulder. Your child may hear some snap, crackle, and pops, which will lessen each time the exercise is repeated.

Yoga

This is another excellent tension reliever. Look for classes specifically designed for children; they're very popular these days.

NOSEBLEEDS

Nosebleeds can be a symptom of many things: allergies, an overly dry environment, a cold, fragile capillaries, high blood pressure, diet. Chronic nosebleeds will need some detective work in order to first determine the cause, and then the solution.

Quick & Easy Remedies

    ☞ To stop light nosebleeds, tear a piece of brown paper from a grocery bag and place it inside the top lip, against the upper gum.

    ☞ Pressing firmly against the lip right under the nose will stimulate an acupressure point that stops bleeding and form a pressure bandage which helps stem the flow of blood.

    ☞ Nosebleeds may be stopped by pinching the nostrils closed for 10 minutes (using the thumb and forefinger of one hand) and breathing through the mouth. Have your child sit slightly forward so the blood doesn't run down the throat.

The Healer of All Healers

To curtail heavy nosebleeds, a dose of cayenne pepper taken internally works beautifully. Cayenne, one of nature's most miraculous healers, dramatically stops bleeding (internal or external) in 10 seconds by equalizing blood pressure. It is high in Vitamin K, which has well-documented clotting properties.

I had long heard of cayenne's ability to stop nosebleeds, but never had the opportunity to see it in action—until the day a teenaged client experienced a heavy nosebleed in my office just as she was describing the problem! I explained the cayenne therapy to her, and she willingly agreed to give it a try. As she was drinking more water to quell cayenne's burning sensation in her throat, we realized the nosebleed had stopped as suddenly as it had started. She, her mother, and I looked at each other with great surprise. Frankly, I had never seen any remedy work quite this fast. Best of all, my client continued to use this treatment and her nosebleeds stopped entirely.

    ☞ Dose according to your child's weight (see Chapter 3: Dosing Guidelines) and administer in liquid-extract form.

    ☞ The only drawback is: no matter how you administer it, cayenne does not go down easily. See Chapter 3: Dosing Guidelines/Cayenne Dosing, for the best way to do it.

As a parent, you'll have to judge your child's maturity level to decide if this remedy is appropriate. Most children are fine with this beginning at age 10, but trust your instincts.

INSECT BITES AND STINGS

Spending time in the great outdoors makes all of us vulnerable to bites and stings. Unless your child is allergic to stinging insects, the standard summertime mosquito bite or less frequent bee sting is irritating but easily treatable. While the usual response is to apply a store-bought product that's full of chemicals (which, in some children, can cause even more irritation to the skin and, worse, adds synthetic chemicals to the bloodstream via absorption through the skin), there are many natural anti-inflammatory herbs that will calm the itch of a bite or pain and swelling of a sting.

Lawns, woods, and meadows can be your natural pharmacy, but you must thoroughly acquaint yourself with these healing plants. Plant identification books are easily obtained in the library or bookstore. Choose a quiet time to familiarize yourself with what is available and appropriate to use, as you will want to be absolutely sure you know how to correctly identify a healing plant (and emergencies are not the time to start doing this). My favorite plant identification book is *A Field Guide to Medicinal Plants: Eastern and Central North America*, by James A. Duke and Steven Foster (Houghton Mifflin, 1992). Some plants that grow in the wild are commercially available at nurseries. Chances are, after you've seen how wondrous their healing properties are, you will want to add these natural healers to your own garden.

Plantain, Comfrey, Chickweed

Commonly found in lawns and woodlands, their leaves' healing action comes alive when the capillary walls are broken down, allowing the juices and their anti-inflammatory benefits to flow.

✿ Use a rock to bruise the ribs and veins in the leaf. Apply to the skin with a bandage.

✿ Or bruise the leaf as I do: chew it up, and it will stick to the skin by itself. (Nature's own bandage!) Actually, the leaves of these plants are sweet and not at all unpleasant to the taste. Allow the leaf poultice to dry on the skin.

✿ Reapply as needed for itch relief.

✿ You must be certain that the area from which you've picked the leaf has not been treated with chemicals.

Aloe

Aloe's soothing, anti-inflammatory properties help relieve itch, pain, and swelling.

✿ Break a stalk of the aloe plant and apply a thick layer of its soothing inner gel to the affected area.

✿ Allow the area to air dry or cover with a bandage.

✿ Reapply as needed.

Lavender

The calming, nervine properties concentrated in the distillation of lavender's essential-oil compounds help to quiet inflamed skin.

✿ Rub a drop or two of the essential oil of the lavender plant on the affected area. This is one of the only essential oils that can be applied to the skin without dilution.

✿ May be reapplied every couple of hours, if needed.

Peppermint

The essential oil of peppermint can help to numb the skin, reducing the itchy sensation.

✿ Apply one drop peppermint oil to the affected area.

❀ It is not necessary to cover the oil. However, if your child touches the spot and then touches his eyes, the peppermint oil may irritate them. Therefore, if your child is not able to refrain from touching the oil, do cover it with a bandage.

Yellow Onion

The onion's detoxifying sulfur compounds help to neutralize the poison of the bite or venom of the sting, reducing inflammation.

❀ To ease the pain and swelling of a sting, apply a ¼" slice of onion, holding it in place with surgical tape, cloth, or bandage. Apply a new slice every couple of hours, if needed.

❀ To relieve the itch of an insect bite, cut an onion open to expose its juicy surface and rub on the bite. *Voilà*—instant itch relief! This remedy can be repeated as often as needed.

Tea Tree Oil

❀ One drop of this potent, detoxifying essential oil is all that is needed to reduce the itch of a bug bite.

❀ If your child finds the tea tree oil too irritating, mix 3 drops tea tree into ½ teaspoon vegetable or nut oil and dab onto itchy bites.

Calendula

Noted for its soothing, anti-inflammatory, and emollient qualities, calendula helps to reduce redness and pain associated with skin swelling.

❀ A gel, lotion, or cream made from calendula flowers can be purchased at most health food stores.

❀ Coat the affected area with a thin layer of the calendula preparation.

❀ Reapply as often as is needed.

Vitamin E

The swelling and inflammation of insect stings can be soothed with the emollient properties of vitamin E.

- ❀ Puncture a capsule with a straight pin and coat the affected area with the oil.
- ❀ Reapply as needed.

Castor Oil

Well respected for its ability to speed up lymphatic flow, thereby dispersing toxins, castor oil quickly relieves pain and swelling.

- ❀ Apply a thin coating of castor oil to your child's insect bite or sting.
- ❀ Reapply as needed.

Dr. Christopher's CMM Ointment

Once again, our friend Dr. Christopher comes to the rescue! The base of this wonderful ointment contains beeswax and olive oil, the latter a soothing emollient. It also contains comfrey, plantain, chickweed, marshmallow root, and mullein, effective anti-inflammatories.

- ❀ Apply a thin coating of the ointment to the affected area.
- ❀ Reapply as needed.

Chamomile Compress

Inflamed skin can be the result of insect bites, heat rash, reaction to skin products, or a simple tussle in the brambles. Chamomile's anti-inflammatory properties reduce itching and irritation.

- ❀ Prepare the tea by steeping 2 teaspoons dried chamomile flowers in 1 cup boiled water until cool. (To hasten the cooling process, add a few ice cubes.)

- ✿ To produce a clear liquid, strain out the herb.
- ✿ Dip a cotton cloth into the tea and apply the chamomile-soaked cloth to the affected area.
- ✿ Cover with plastic wrap to keep the compress moist and to prevent it from dripping.
- ✿ Reapply every 2–4 hours, if needed.
- ✿ For a more concentrated treatment, instead of straining out the flowers, pack them onto the skin with the soaked cotton cloth. Cover with plastic to keep moist.

For your herbal enlightenment, the cloth dipped into the strained-tea infusion is called a compress; with the steeped flowers, it becomes a poultice. I know this word sounds quite ancient, but a poultice is merely a moist mass of herbs applied externally. (See the section on Applications for more information.)

At the same time, if the inflammation is causing upset in your little one, you can dilute ¼ cup of the chamomile tea with a little water, sweeten with honey, and serve up a soothing drink that is sure to calm his stomach and emotions.

Baking Soda

The minerals in a paste of baking soda and water provide soothing, quick relief from pain and inflammation.

- ✿ In the palm of your hand or, if you prefer, in a small dish, put a teaspoon of baking soda.
- ✿ Moisten with just enough water to make a paste.
- ✿ Apply to affected area, covering with gauze and surgical tape.
- ✿ Reapply every couple of hours, as needed.

Mud

The Aztecs knew it, now so do you: the minerals in a mud pack provide instant, on-the-spot relief from the pain and inflammation of a bite or sting.

  ⚘ To a handful of soil add just enough water to make a paste.

  ⚘ Apply to affected area, reapplying as often as is necessary for relief.

Banana

If the stinger of a bee or wasp remains embedded in your child's skin, the enzymes in a ripened banana peel will draw the stinger to the surface for easy removal.

  ⚘ Cut a 1" square piece of ripened banana peel to cover the affected area.

  ⚘ Apply the pulp side of the banana peel against the skin.

  ⚘ Hold the banana peel in place with a piece of surgical tape. (See Appendix A for a description of the type of surgical tape I have found to work best.)

  ⚘ Leave on overnight. In the morning, the banana will have drawn the foreign matter to the surface, ready for easy removal—or, better still, may show in the peel when you remove it from the skin. More tenacious stingers may require one or two more nights of this treatment, in which case you should use a fresh section of peel each time.

Apis

If your child has a life-threatening anaphylactic reaction to stinging insects (when the throat begins to swell), you must get her to the emergency room right away. If you have been prepared for this sting-ing insect allergy, you may already have a medical kit for emergency treatment. In addition to the medical treatment, whether at home or on the way to the hospital, you can give her a homeopathic remedy called apis. If you know your child has a stinging insect allergy, it would be wise to keep this remedy on hand at all times.

  ⚘ Purchase the apis in 30c potency from a health food store or pharmacy.

✿ To administer, place two of the sweet-tasting pellets under your child's tongue and let dissolve.

✿ If necessary, this dose can be repeated every 10–15 minutes until your child is breathing better or receives medical attention. If your infant or child is too young to dissolve pellets under the tongue, see Appendix G for a resource for ordering apis in liquid form.

✿ Homeopathic remedies are fragile substances that can easily be antidoted by the oils in your skin so do not handle them. Instead, tap the dose into the vial's cap and transfer into your child's mouth.

Be Fragrance Free

Always keep in mind that insects like sweet smells, so it would be wise to refrain from using any fragranced product on your child at those times of the year when insects are prevalent—or, of course, if you're traveling to an insect-prone area.

It would be best if people in the company of your child would also refrain from wearing scented products so as not to draw insects into your child's immediate environment. Shampoo, soap, perfume, after shave, suntan lotion, and even scented lip gloss attract bugs!

A Word About Insect Repellents

Commercial bug repellents contain chemicals that may irritate skin and, worse, their toxic residues can wind up in the liver and bloodstream.

There are many natural bug-repellent preparations, but I wouldn't want to be around you if you were using them because I don't like how they smell! A pleasant alternative is the essential oil of pennyroyal. Included in the medicinal repertoire of a variety of cultures for thousands of years, it has a refreshingly minty aroma and, most importantly, contains naturally occurring chemicals loathed by mosquitoes.

Many of my clients send their children to summer camp with this pennyroyal mosquito repellent and, as a result, other campers and their counselors happily benefit as well. I have even used this successfully in the densely mosquito-infested Everglades.

Pennyroyal Mosquito Repellent

   ❋ Mix 10 drops oil of pennyroyal with 1 ounce almond oil for a fragrant and extremely effective mosquito repellent.

   ❋ Dab the oil on your child's wrists, ankles, neck, and hair.

   ❋ Reapply every 2–4 hours, as needed.

A last word about insect bites: according to Dr. Peter D'Adamo, author of *Eat Right for Your Blood Type* (Putnam, 1996), scientific literature reveals that people with type A blood are more likely to attract biting bugs than folks with other blood types. Perhaps this is why biting bugs find me so delectable!

LYME DISEASE

Named for the town of East Lyme, CT, where the pathogen was first identified, a Lyme-infected tick, as it feeds off its host, passes a spirochete, a bacterial microorganism, into the bloodstream.

Supporting the Body. When a child is quickly treated with an antibiotic for Lyme disease, the result is usually a swift and positive healing. The antibiotic, designed to attack bacteria, does not differentiate between beneficial and harmful bacteria and may deplete the good bacteria located in the intestinal tract. I recommend the addition of acidophilus (see page 210 for description and dosing suggestions) to prevent an occurrence of candida from the antibiotic. I also suggest giving your child echinacea. It supports the immune system which can be depleted by antibiotic use.

The Viral Connection. When my son, Chris, had Lyme disease, blood tests confirmed that it was accompanied by the virulent bacteria ehrlichiosis, so his doctor immediately put him on an antibiotic.

In addition to the natural supports, acidophilus and echinacea, I gave him homeopathic remedies to deal with the particular strains of virus that kinesiologically tested as piggybacking the spirochete (which I have found to be quite common in the Northeast area of the United States). I have consistently found that when children (and adults) do not recover quickly with antibiotic therapy, it may be because viruses are involved—and, as you may know, viruses do not respond to antibiotics. They do, however, respond quite nicely to specific homeopathics that can be given at the same time as antibiotics—without interfering with each other.

Locating a Health Practitioner. If your child's Lyme disease is not responding well to the antibiotics alone, you may wish to consult with a health practitioner who works with disease-specific homeopathics and who is familiar with the viruses that are known to attach themselves to the ticks that transfer this disease. In fact, if your child has been bitten by a tick in an area where Lyme disease is prevalent (while on vacation, at camp, etc.), I recommend seeking help from a practitioner in that locale rather than in your home town, especially if Lyme disease is not a common problem where you live. To locate a health-care practitioner in your area, specializing in these Lyme-related remedies, contact Healers Who Share, 303-428-4584.

Eating Healthfully. While your child's body is dealing with the foreign invaders, you should reduce her sugar intake to avoid its additional burden to the immune system, and see that she eats especially nutritious foods so as not to pose any additional challenges to the body at this time.

JELLYFISH STINGS

My co-writer, David, wishes he'd known about this remedy when he was at summer camp on the Chesapeake Bay, where the jellyfish found him ever so sweet a treat. The excellent *Natural Health* magazine, available in health food stores and by subscription, reports that jellyfish stings will be aggravated if washed in fresh water. Instead, bathe the affected area in vinegar, an antimicrobial, which helps to neutralize toxins by reestablishing pH, the body's acid/alkaline balance.

- ❀ Using a cotton ball, soak the area well with apple cider vinegar.
- ❀ After soaking, thickly cover the area with a paste made with four parts flour, one part salt, and water. This is a drawing paste to help pull out toxins.
- ❀ Cover with roller gauze and surgical tape, and your child should feel relief within an hour.
- ❀ Because the paste can be difficult to remove, it may need to be soaked with water first.

POISON IVY

Catch That Dot

When my poison-ivy-sensitive sons recognize the first "dot" or two of the dreaded rash, they are able to stop the reaction from going any further if they take action right away.

- ❀ The homeopathic preparation, Rhus. Tox., is an extremely dilute form of the poison ivy toxin. While it may sound a little scary to be giving your child that which he is reacting to, keep in mind that is exactly what is done with allergy injections. This is recognized around the world as a very safe remedy as long as it is used properly.
- ❀ Homeopathic pellets cannot be handled because the oils in the skin will antidote their fragile components; therefore, tap the dose into the plastic cap that is provided and drop it under your child's tongue to dissolve. Your child won't mind—it tastes sweet. As with all homeopathic remedies, no food or drink can be ingested 20 minutes before and 20 minutes after taking the remedy.

   ❀ Take 2 pellets of homeopathic Rhus. Tox. (available in health food stores, and now in many pharmacies, as well), potency 30c.

   ❀ Repeat the dose 2–3 more times that day.

Dry It Up

If the rash is already in an advanced stage, head for the pharmacy and purchase a product called Domeboro (a boric acid solution) in powdered form. By neutralizing the poison ivy toxin, it diminishes the itch, dries up the oozing, and relieves inflammation within hours. When one of my sons, Chris, was little, and before I was aware of Rhus. Tox., I used to keep long strips of a torn-up sheet for the sole purpose of compressing Domeboro. He'd lie in front of the TV for the healing sessions, and by the next day, even the worst rashes were vastly improved.

   ❀ Dissolve two packets in a pint of lukewarm water.

   ❀ Dip a cotton cloth into the solution, and compress the sites of the rash for 20 minutes, 3 times a day.

HERBAL FIRST AID KIT

As a parent, you wouldn't dream of going on a trip—or maybe even a day's outing—without a first aid kit, and with good reason. After all, where there are kids, there are minor mishaps, and it's the mark of a concerned caregiver to be prepared at all times.

So why not assemble an herbal first aid kit? It inspires confidence, at least for me, and I wouldn't dream of going on even a short trip without one. Just think of all the little things that transpire to make a child (and you) feel miserable, and you'll agree on the importance of this herbal kit.

First aid does not have to mean something serious. Rather, it can just mean the "first" thing you would use to "aid" the problem at hand. Doesn't this make it seem less intimidating?

Personalize Your Kit

To create a first aid kit that is personalized to your children's needs, sit down and think of the problems to which they are prone. If earaches are never an issue for your children (as they weren't for mine), then you needn't include herbs to combat this problem. If, on the other hand, cuts and scrapes seem to love your child, or if nasal congestion is a recurrent issue, herbs to treat these should certainly be included in your first aid kit.

I suggest reviewing sections of this book for the discomforts common to your child as a means of creating a list of remedies that you can feasibly include in your personal kit. Be on the lookout for remedies that do double duty; many herbs are versatile enough to be used for more than one problem.

Keep the Kit Portable

Maybe it's because I'm so often lecturing on the road, but I have a thing about packing as lightly as possible, either for a big trip or a single day's outing. I've discovered that sample-sized perfume vials are the perfect vessel for carrying a single dose of a liquid extract or essential oils.

Film canisters make handy containers for small amounts of dried herbs, ointments, and oils; so do sample cosmetic containers. Jewelers' plastic zip pouches are great for capsules and dried herbs. Whatever clever packaging you devise, be sure to clean it thoroughly of its previous contents.

Standard First Aid Supplies

To keep your kit as compact as possible, the supplies you use should be versatile. Mine includes the following:

❀ Roller gauze and a small roll of surgical tape. These can be used creatively to cover any type of bleeding injury as well as hold a poultice in place. Think you would never need a poul-

tice for a day trip? How about something as simple but annoy-
ing (and, sometimes, downright painful) as a splinter? Of
course you won't be carrying a banana peel in your first aid kit,
but there are supermarkets everywhere, and with the help of
roller gauze and surgical tape, you'll be able to affix the peel to
the affected area.

❖ A miniature penknife for cutting bandages, scooping herbal
preparations from their containers, mixing preparations, etc.

❖ A straight pin is a helpful item to have in your kit so that you
can puncture the vitamin E capsule you could include.

Andrea's First Aid Kit

As an example, I'll review remedies I've had in my first aid kits over
the years. Keep in mind, I keep mine small for easy portability. For
this reason, I prefer to keep powdered echinacea for its versatility, as
opposed to the liquid extract and then add water, if needed. (I never
leave home without a ½-ounce dropper bottle of echinacea in my
handbag anyway.) You may be happy with a kit that contains ½-
ounce dropper bottles (see Appendix G for resources) of prepared
extracts. Please note that each of these herbs is discussed more fully
in its appropriate section elsewhere in this book.

❖ **Powdered cayenne,** known as the herbalist's first aid herb, can
be used externally for bleeding cuts or internally for sinus
headaches, asthma attacks, to stop nosebleeds, or to revive
your child from a fainting spell.

❖ **Powdered echinacea** can be applied dry to cuts and wounds,
hydrated with water or juice, and given at the first sign of a
cold or whatever seems to be causing your child to be out of
sorts. My philosophy is this: when in doubt, give echinacea.
Our immune systems can always use a little boost!

❖ **Dr. Christopher's SHA** comes in capsule or liquid form and
is great for what its letters stand for: sinus, hay fever, and
allergy.

❀ **Peppermint oil** can be put in water to sip and inhale for digestive upset, nausea, headache, sinus congestion. Simply inhaling it straight from the bottle will help headache, sinuses, and nausea. A tiny bit can be applied to the temples for headache, as well.

❀ **Ginger powder** can be mixed with water (or you can include ginger capsules in your kit) for motion sickness, as well as digestive upsets.

❀ **Dr. Christopher's BF&C** ointment can be used for all sorts of skin itches and irritations, bumps, and bruises, even for chapped lips. You can transfer just a little from its original container into an old lip-gloss pot for your first aid kit.

❀ **Aloe gel** can calm a burn, skin irritation, or sunburn.

❀ **Castor oil** can be used immediately after a vaccination, on a bruise or irritated skin, on insect bites, and stings.

❀ **Vitamin E** is good for minor burns, insect bites, and stings.

❀ **Mullein oil** can be dropped into the ear at the first sign of trouble or applied to a scrape.

❀ **Garlic oil** can be dropped into the ear, along with mullein oil, if you suspect infection. It can also be given internally, along with echinacea for anything about to become a something!

❀ **Bach Flower Rescue Remedy** can be used for all sorts of emotional issues. It can provide your child with emotional support due to a physical trauma or restore equilibrium in a toy store tantrum.

❀ **Cell salts** come in travel-size cases that are fine for overnight trips or they can be left in the trunk of your car; but strictly speaking, these do not qualify as mini–travel kit components. I do, however, include vials of one or two of the salts I use most often. For example, Calc. Sulph. is terrific for sore throats.

❀ **Acidophilus** capsules are easy to include and come in handy if the stomach is "off" in one way or another.

❀ **Dr. Christopher's Fen LB** (lower bowel) comes with me whenever I take a trip. Many people find that traveling can cause the bowels to go off schedule, and this herbal combination is excellent for constipation. It comes in capsule and liquid form. See Appendix G for resources, or check this formula's ingredients in Appendix H and select a similar product from the health food store.

- ❀ **Nervine formula.** Sleep patterns are often disturbed while traveling. A formula containing nervine herbs such as valerian, passionflower, and hops helps provide a good night's sleep.
- ❀ **Keeping your kit fresh.** Periodically review the freshness of your kit's herbs. Herbs exposed to heat and humidity may lose their potency faster than those stored properly at home (see p. 216 for storage guidelines). Determine freshness by taste, appearance, and smell.

Once you've assembled your first aid kit, you'll see how very different it is from the standard version. Your kit will be so versatile that you'll be ready to help everyone around you.

First Aid Home Herbal Pack

At some point during my travels, I came across a soothing herbal pack that can almost always be relied on to make the "hurt" go away. It's somewhat like a beanbag, filled instead with fragrant healing herbs that help relieve sundry aches and pains, soothe nerves, and even calm a headache. Nature's Therapy Herb Pac (see Appendix G for resources) comes in assorted fabrics, many especially designed to appeal to children.

- ❀ Store the pack in the freezer. As a cold application, it's perfect for insect stings, shinbone pain, sunburn, headaches, swelling from injury—wherever you would normally use an ice pack. Alternate on and off every 5–10 minutes.
- ❀ For a warm application, heat in a microwave or conventional oven set at 200 degrees. It can help relieve the stress of sports injuries, tense muscles, cramps, sinusitis, and colicky tummy. You can also use it as a toasty security blanket to soothe a sagging spirit and ease a little one to sleep. The pack can stay in place until it cools. Rewarm as needed.

5

The Upper Respiratory System

Statistics indicate that the average American schoolchild has several colds a year. Comforted—falsely—by statistics, parents accept all manner of cold and flu as "normal childhood diseases." "After all," we tell ourselves, "it could be worse. What's a case of the sniffles or the odd ear infection now and then? It's something all kids need to go through."

This is erroneous thinking. Health, not sickness, is the body's normal state of being. Just because all the other kids at school are sick doesn't mean yours have to be. You can maintain a respectable level of wellness for your child even in the face of the nastiest colds and flu.

Herbs are especially useful in healing flare-ups of the upper respiratory system. Many of the therapies I present here are preventative so the old adage that "all kids get sick" doesn't have to prove true in your home—it certainly didn't in mine.

SORE THROATS

Gargle Without the Giggle

Gargles are an age-old method of bringing soothing substances to sore throats. To see if your child is capable of gargling liquids:

⚕ Have her hold a small mouthful of plain water towards the back of the throat.
⚕ If this is easily done, gargling can become a fun activity by vocalizing, causing the liquid to vibrate. Be careful, though, too much fun can cause giggling, which can turn gargling into choking.
⚕ If vocalizing makes your child uncomfortable, simply have her retain the liquid in the throat while you count, encouraging her to hold it a moment longer.
⚕ Be sure the liquid is expectorated (spat out) so the toxins drawn out from the swollen tissue are not swallowed.

Salty Lemon Gargle

The astringent properties of lemon juice and common table salt (or, for a more pure version, sea salt, found in all health food stores), when combined with warm water and used as a gargle, shrink swollen tissue. As a result, this classic blend reduces the inflammation and pain of sore throats while providing excellent antimicrobial protection.

⚕ Combine the juice of half a lemon with one tablespoon salt in ½ cup warm water.
⚕ Have your child gargle with this mixture at least four times a day.
⚕ To further enhance the astringency and antimicrobial action of this gargle, mix the lemon and salt into ½ cup sage tea instead of plain water. See Appendix A for directions for preparing the herb tea.

Grapefruit Seed Gargle

The extract of the grapefruit seed contains potent antimicrobial as well as astringent constituents that help relieve an inflamed, sore throat.

⚕ Add 4–6 drops grapefruit seed extract (purchased in health food stores) to ½ glass water.

❧ Have your child gargle with the diluted extract, spitting it out after each gargle.

Throat-Healing Herbs

In addition to the herbs you would give for a cold, a sore throat may be comforted with:

❧ Slippery elm lozenges (available at health food stores). Slippery elm is an herb with soothing, anti-inflammatory properties.

❧ A diluted spray of echinacea and goldenseal, sprayed on the back of the throat. To make this antimicrobial spray, dilute 10 drops of each herb in 4 ounces of water.

❧ A spoonful of honey which is anti-inflammatory as well as anti-microbial is a traditional remedy for soothing the throats of opera singers before performances. Your child can lick the honey right off the spoon to experience its soothing properties as it slides down her irritated throat.

❧ A room vaporizer containing eucalyptus oil. The vaporizer's hydrating mist soothes a dry, irritated throat while the eucalyptus emits its antimicrobial properties into the surrounding air.

❧ A tea/gargle of the soothing, anti-inflammatory herbs licorice root and slippery elm bark (see Appendix A for directions for preparing a decoction).

❧ A gargle with sage or raspberry leaf tea, effective astringents, can help reduce the swollen tissue of a sore throat.

EAR INFECTIONS

Medical statistics tell us that 75% of children have at least three ear infections before the age of six. What's more, most of us either have or know a child who repeatedly suffers from what we have tacitly come to accept as a common childhood illness. Doesn't it make you wonder why, with all the advances of modern medicine, children seem to suffer from ear infections more, rather than less often, than they did even 20 years ago?

Antibiotics: The Culprit or the Cure? I believe the chronic use of antibiotics is more than partly to blame. Many doctors inform frustrated parents that their infants suffer from ear maladies because they were born with narrowed Eustachian tubes (more on this later). The children are then put on one or more cycles of antibiotics in an attempt to rid the ear of recurring infections. Some children respond well; others are put on a round-robin of antibiotic treatments (sometimes for years); and others still require surgery. A study reported in a 1991 edition of the *Journal of the American Medical Association* found that children given an antibiotic for ear infections were two to six times more likely to develop a recurrence than children who did not receive the antibiotic treatment. Also, the recurrent infections caused an increase in impaired hearing due to scar tissue from the repeated incidents. Often, the impaired hearing is the cause of delayed speech.

Over $3.5 billion is spent by American parents every year on the treatment of ear infections, primarily on antibiotics. I am not the only one asking the question: What long-term effects do antibiotics have on developing immune systems? Medical researchers are still debating this issue, but I believe from empirical evidence that the long-term use of antibiotics can have definite deleterious effects on our bodies—and this is even more pronounced when we consider that children's immune systems are still immature. This is yet another compelling reason why natural healing has taken (and will continue to take) North America by storm.

Narrowed Eustachian Tubes and Our Toxic Environment I find it hard to accept that the human reproductive system has so dramatically biodiversified in the last 20 years that we now birth children with "narrowed Eustachian tubes." Rather, I believe that the narrowing of these inner-ear conduits is an inflammatory response to substances that offend children's bodies.

In the case of newborns, all kinds of environmental factors can take their toll on the infant's immune system. The great French writer Antoine de St.-Exupéry *(The Little Prince)* wrote aphoristically of the power of anticipation, and what human event can begin to equal the arrival of a new baby? We parents take special care to ensure that baby's nursery is cheery, safe, and warm, but fail to take into account the array of possible irritants. Just think—the typical nursery contains new carpeting, paint, furniture, linens, curtains, and stuffed animals. What do we have here? Although it's quite the opposite of what you would ever want for baby, it's nothing short of a mini-chemical factory!

Some infants' immune systems will be able to handle the chemical onslaught. Others, depending upon their genetic predisposition, may respond with asthma, skin afflictions, ear infections, or some other challenge to their immature immune systems. In the case of ear infections, the Eustachian tubes may narrow as an inflammatory response to these toxic substances. The narrowed tubes may cause a backup of fluids and consequently become infected. Most physicians prescribe antibiotics without ever addressing the root cause of these narrowed ear tubes.

In the last 10 years, billions of gallons of poisonous chemicals have been dumped into our waterways, pumped into the air we breathe, and integrated into the farming, manufacturing, and transport of the foods we eat.

So What's a Parent to Do? So what's a parent to do? Take charge of what you *can* take charge of. Make sure the nursery is the safest possible environment: dust-and chemical-free. Wash all clothes and linens before putting them near baby's skin. Use the most natural products you can find on your child's body, and be sure they are fragrance-free.

Kinesiologically test (see the Appendix C on food testing) every food your child ingests, because poorly tolerated foods can result in the buildup of mucus, which is a precursor to many ear infections. The nursing mother can be tested, as well, for the foods she is passing on to her baby. Foods that are the most common offenders include dairy, soy, wheat, corn, peanuts, chocolate, orange juice, and eggs.

Diet, Herbs, and Chiropractic

The key word is prevention. But what if ear infections are already a recurrent problem in your child's life? I recommend the following courses of action at the earliest signs of ear discomfort:

- ❧ Limit the intake of sugar. Processed sugar is a challenge to the body and feeds fungal, parasitic, and bacterial infections.
- ❧ Eliminate milk and cheese from the diet. Dairy can be a mucus-forming food, and your child is already exhibiting difficulty in handling mucus, so it's wise not to create any added burdens at this time. (Yogurt, however, is often well tolerated.)
- ❧ Dose your child with echinacea at the first sign of infection. Colds usually wind up in the ears of children predisposed to weakness in this part of their body. If you can prevent a cold from blossoming, you will have prevented another ear infection from developing. See section on colds for instructions on how to administer echinacea and the herbs described below.
- ❧ If a cold does take hold, introduce an herbal decongestant, making sure your child takes it four times a day. These can be found in any health food store.
- ❧ Add garlic to your child's diet. Garlic is naturally antibacterial, as well as antifungal, antiviral, and antiparasitic. A fresh clove can be chopped into mashed potatoes or put on toast with butter. Older children can take garlic in tablet form, and younger kids can easily take oil of garlic. Whatever form you choose, be sure your child has garlic three times a day.
- ❧ If infected fluid has settled in the ear, and there is no perforation of the eardrum (check with your physician to be sure of this), put a drop or two of antimicrobial garlic oil in each ear, along with a drop or two of oil of mullein flower.

Mullein flower is well known for its anti-inflammatory, decongestant action in the ear. I do not, however, recommend the purchase of the combination garlic/mullein oil that many health food stores carry because garlic oil *can* be ingested, while oil of mullein *cannot*. Buy them separately and combine, if needed, for application in the ear. The easiest time to administer eardrops is when a child is sleeping.

- ✿ If there is pain accompanying fluid in the ear, add a drop or two of St. John's Wort oil to the above oils. Its ability to calm nerve sensitivity may help to diminish the discomfort.

- ✿ For many children, chiropractic adjustments have been instrumental in preventing recurrent ear infections. The field of chiropractic focuses on subluxations, vertebrae (spinal bones) that are out of alignment. If there is a misalignment in the area of spinal nerves leading to the ears, it is possible that ear problems could be helped by the increased blood-and-oxygen flow of a corrected subluxation.

Take Charge and Be Vigilant! As a final word, vigilance is absolutely key. If you are prepared to take charge of your child's ear infections using natural methods, be certain that the condition is improving; otherwise, get medical help. But don't be afraid to take charge by implementing all of the above protocols even while your child is on an antibiotic. I have seen even the most chronic ear infections turned around, indeed eliminated, from a child's life by using the programs outlined above.

EARACHES

The Onion Pain Reliever

The common, yellow onion is high in antimicrobial compounds, reduces swelling, and promotes circulation.

To reduce or eliminate pain in the ear:

- Cut a yellow onion in half and warm it in the oven at 200 degrees for a few minutes.
- Wrap the warmed onion in cheesecloth and hold against the child's ear until the onion has cooled.
- The wrapped onion can be reheated in the oven and used repeatedly.

Cell Salt Therapy

For a complete description of cell salts and dosing instructions for these pleasant-tasting and easily administered substances, see Appendix F. *The Biochemic Handbook* describes the following cell salts as especially helpful in both eliminating ear maladies and helping ease the symptoms:

Ferr. Phos. For inflammatory earache with burning, throbbing pain, especially after exposure to cold or wet weather.
Kali Mur. For earache with swelling of the Eustachian tubes or catarrhal inflammation of the middle ear.
Nat. Mur. For roaring in the ears, along with dullness of hearing and watering of the ear.
Kali Phos. For dullness of hearing and noises in the head, plus accompanying nervous symptoms.
Calc. Sulph. Discharges from the ear, sometimes mixed with blood.

ITCHY EARS

Tea Tree and Garlic

If your child's ears do not respond well to the following suggestions and tend to be chronically itchy, then an internal yeast/fungal infection should be considered as a probable cause. In this case, itchy ears will clear up without anything being applied topically by clearing the systemic fungus with remedies taken internally. See p. 209 for guidelines for fungal infections.

Itchy ears may be symptomatic of a bacteria, fungus, or parasite. In any case, I have found the oil of the Australian tea tree (easily found in health food stores) to be an easy solution.

- ❧ Simply moisten a cotton swab with tea tree oil and dab on the affected areas, morning and night.
- ❧ If your child finds the pure tea tree oil too irritating, dilute it with a mild vegetable or nut oil like sunflower, almond, or olive by adding 3 drops tea tree oil to ½–1 teaspoon of the carrier oil.
- ❧ Keep in mind that sugar feeds these microorganisms, so keep your child's diet as sugar-free as possible, at least until the itchiness clears up.
- ❧ If more help is needed, put two drops garlic oil (readily available in health food stores) into both ears, as long as there is no perforation of the eardrum. (A medical examination would reveal this.) Both tea tree oil and garlic oil treatments can be used concurrently. After both applications, plug the ear with cotton.

WAXY BUILD-UP

Peppermint De-Clogger

Warmed oil of peppermint diluted in olive oil at bedtime should correct this problem.

- ❧ Combine 2 drops oil of peppermint with ½ teaspoon olive oil in a small glass.
- ❧ To warm the oils, place bottom of glass in a small bowl of hot water for a few minutes.
- ❧ While your child is sleeping, draw the oil mixture up into an eye dropper and insert as much oil as the ear will hold without overflowing.

❀ Plug the ear with a piece of cotton. Even though the cotton will absorb some of it, the oil will remain effectively localized.
❀ Again, keep in mind that oils cannot be inserted into an ear with a perforated eardrum.

EYE IRRITATIONS

When eyes are red, sore, or irritated as a result of allergies, environmental pollutants, or fatigue, the anti-inflammatory properties of calendula and chamomile provide gentle relief in the form of compresses or eyedrops.

Calendula/Chamomile Eye Therapy Compress

❀ Boil 1 cup steam-distilled water (available in health food stores or supermarkets) and pour over 2 teaspoons dried calendula flowers or dried chamomile flowers.
❀ Steep until just warm, and strain.
❀ Dip a washcloth or cotton pads in the tea, squeezing gently; then apply over eyelids for 20 minutes.
❀ Repeat 3–4 times a day, reheating the tea for a more soothing effect. The tea may be stored in the refrigerator for 3 days.

Calendula/Chamomile Eyedrop Therapy

❀ Prepare the tea infusion as for the compress above and let cool.
❀ Strain fluid very well through layers of cheesecloth, a linen napkin, or a paper coffee filter.
❀ Pour into a dropper bottle, administering 1–2 drops in each eye, 3 to 4 times daily. The eye drops are good for three days if stored in the refrigerator.

Dr. John R. Christopher, lovingly known as the father of modern-day herbalism, created a wonderful formula for the eyes that can be found in health food stores everywhere (or see Appendix G for ordering information). These eye drops help heal conjunctivitis (pinkeye), sties, crustiness, discharges, and any other situation that requires cleansing of the eye tissue. It is important to know that this remedy may draw out toxins from the eyes. Thus, do not be alarmed if yellow or green mucus starts to run from your child's eyes as a result of this therapy. There is a dash of cayenne in the formula which may cause a momentary sting, but the results will be well worth it, as the continued use of this eye solution will help clear up problems long-term.

Dr. Christopher's Herbal Eyebright Formula

This formula contains encapsulated herbs that are antimicrobial, anti-inflammatory, cleansing, and nourishing to the eyes—bayberry bark, eyebright herb, goldenseal root, raspberry leaf, and cayenne.*

- ❀ Open one capsule into ⅓ cup boiled distilled water. Steep until cool.
- ❀ Thoroughly strain through layered cheesecloth, linen napkin, or paper coffee filter until liquid is clear, then pour into an eyedropper bottle.
- ❀ Put 2 drops of the formula in each eye 3 times a day. Eye drops will last 3 days in your refrigerator.

As a parent, my experience with this formula has been that major improvement can be expected within 3 days. In accordance with Andrea's Rule of Three (see page 3), seek medical attention if you do not see a marked change for the better by then.

---

*If your child just cannot tolerate the brief sting of the cayenne, you may prepare our own version of this formula without this herb by purchasing the dried, cut herbs separately and decocting the bayberry bark and goldenseal root together, steeping the raspberry leaf and eyebright together (see Appendix A for directions for preparing the teas), then combining the two liquids to make the eyedrops.

DIGESTIVE HEADACHES

Often, a headache can be related to something your child has eaten. Eight-year-old Josh developed a stomachache and headache shortly after lunch. At the end of the school day, he wasn't feeling up to attending his after-school activity; since his mother had not yet arrived at home, he came to visit with me.

"Can I give you something that would help take away your headache and stomachache?" I asked Josh. "Oh, no," he replied. "My mother told me never to take medicine from anyone." "Well, how about a cup of peppermint tea?" I offered. "Oh, that would be good," said Josh—and a half-hour later, he was feeling just fine.

Soothing Peppermint Tea #1

Peppermint's essential oil contains antispasmodic and digestive properties, the perfect combination to relieve a headache and stomachache.

- ❀ Steep 1 teaspoon peppermint leaves in one cup boiled water for 15 minutes, keeping the cup covered in order to retain the potency of the essential oil contained in the leaves.
- ❀ Strain and serve with honey, if desired. Honey, known for its anti-inflammatory properties, can also help soothe an upset stomach.

Soothing Peppermint Tea #2

- ❀ Add one drop (not two!) oil of peppermint to one cup warm water.
- ❀ Add honey, and serve immediately.

The leaf infusion #1 has a milder, sweeter taste than #2. However, I prefer #2 because its benefits can be enjoyed so quickly. There is, as you can see, no steeping time when you use the essential oil. With either tea, I suggest you have your child sip the beverage with eyes closed, since the essential oil of peppermint may cause tearing (especially if it is of good quality). Inhaling the tea as it is sipped will serve to enhance its many healing benefits.

More Headache-Relieving Remedies

❀ Digestive headaches may also respond well to other gentle, digestive teas such as chamomile or fennel seed.

❀ Acidophilus (see pages 209–210) or plain yogurt (with active cultures) drizzled with honey can help digestive headaches by balancing your child's intestinal flora. Either may be given 3–4 times a day.

❀ Constipation-related headache may be remedied with a dose of a lower-bowel tonic (see Appendix H for ingredients and Appendix G for resources); give it to your child with lots of water.

SINUS-RELATED HEADACHES

There are several effective approaches for headaches related to sinus congestion.

Decongesting Herbs

❀ Have your child inhale the oils of peppermint or eucalyptus for their ability to stimulate mucus secretions.

❀ Prepare the inhalation by adding 1 drop of either essential oil to 1 cup warm water. Have your child close his eyes while he deeply breathes over the cup.

❀ A drop or two of the above oils may be mixed with 1 teaspoon nut or seed oil, such as almond, peach kernel, or grapeseed, and applied to the temples and sinus areas along the cheekbones and across the forehead. This is another way to experience an herbal inhalation. (See figure #1.)

❀ Dilute several drops of a liquid herbal decongestant (found in

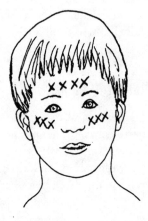

health food stores) in an ounce or two of water or juice. Have your child drink the decongestant every few hours.

✿ Add several drops oil of eucalyptus directly to the bathwater. Have your child breathe deeply while bathing for 10–15 minutes.

✿ Make a compress of peppermint or eucalyptus oils by soaking a washcloth in 3 drops of either essential oil, diluted in 1 cup warm water, and compress to your child's forehead for five to ten minutes.

EMOTIONALLY BASED HEADACHES

The anticipation of an upsetting event (a school exam or dental visit, for example) can precipitate a headache. Give any one or combination of the following remedies to find just the right one to restore your child's spirits.

Lovely Lavender

The essential oil of lavender's calming compounds can be:

✿ Applied undiluted to your child's temples by gently massaging in a drop or two.

❀ Compressed to the forehead (using 3–5 drops in 1 cup warm water).

❀ Put on a tissue, handkerchief, or pillowcase (just a few drops will suffice) and inhaled.

❀ Added to the child's bath water (4–6 drops).

Spirit Soothers

Children's headaches of all kinds respond well to:

❀ The calming effects of the Bach Flower Essence, Rescue Remedy. (See Appendix I for a description.) A few drops added to ½ cup warm water may be patted on the forehead.

❀ Nervine herbs have a calming effect on the muscles and nervous system. When the headache is related to nervous tension, several drops of a nervine formula containing relaxing herbs like valerian, passionflower, hops, oats, diluted in 2 ounces of water or juice will soothe and calm your child.

❀ Chamomile is well known for its relaxing properties. This herb may bring headache relief in the form of a tea or bath.

Chamomile Bath

This wonderful bath can be prepared in one of two ways.

❀ The first method is to add a quart of chamomile tea to the bath water (infusing the flowers as you would for a tea, but doubling the proportions to 2 teaspoons per cup) and steeping twice as long (30 minutes).

The other way to prepare this bath is to turn your bathtub into an oversized teacup!

❀ Fill a muslin bag or a washcloth tied closed with a rubber band with fresh or dried chamomile flowers. If you know of a safe place to pick fresh chamomile flowers, the activity of walking, seeking out the plant, and inhaling its flowers will probably relieve your child's headache! The bath will then be a soothing treat.

 ❀ Suspend the bag or washcloth from the bathtub's faucet so that it is soaking in the bath water as the tub fills.
 ❀ Your child can also rub the chamomile pouch all over her body to derive further benefit from its relaxing properties through skin absorption.

FEVER-RELATED HEADACHES

Fever-Reducing Herbs

Yarrow and elderflower are known as diaphoretic herbs. They encourage sweating which is a good way of releasing toxins from the body.

 ❀ Following Appendix A directions for making herbal infusions, prepare a diaphoretic tea using either or both of the above herbs.
 ❀ Drinking, compressing, or bathing in the teas helps to pull toxins from the body, thereby relieving your child's headache. It helps the healing process when your child joins in deciding whether a tea, compress, or bath (or combination) would be best.

Headache Imagery

Every color vibrates to its own frequency or wave of energy. Color visualization can often defuse a headache by combining the quieting activity of imagery with the calming vibrations of certain colors.

 ❀ With his eyes closed, ask your child to picture the color blue in his mind. (Blue represents a cool, calm sensation.) Your child may see this color as a blue sky, or he may see himself floating on a blue cloud.

❧ Have him slowly and deeply breathe in the color blue and, as he slowly exhales, see the "toxins" of the headache leaving the body in the form of gray smoke.

❧ Help him to breathe slowly and rhythmically by breathing with him.

This relaxing, nurturing experience can really help a child release the discomfort of a headache. For more information on visualization see Appendix E.

NASAL CONGESTION

Eucalyptus is secretomotory, a stimulator of secretions, which makes it a great herb for decongesting the sinus passages. Whether this condition is caused by allergies or by a cold that's clogging your child's head, a eucalyptus inhaler can bring relief. It is safe and easy to self-administer, so you can send one to school in your child's backpack.

The Eucalyptus Inhaler

❧ Fill a plastic vial with cotton. Add a few drops of oil of eucalyptus, replacing the cap.

❧ Each time your child needs help to breathe, the cap can be removed and a deep inhalation taken from the vial.

The Eucalyptus Vapor

❧ You can fill your child's room with the benefits of eucalyptus by putting several drops oil of eucalyptus in a vaporizer.

The Eucalyptus Bath

❧ Add several drops oil of eucalyptus to the bath water.

❧ Encourage your child to breathe deeply while bathing.

The Eucalyptus Dot

Eucalyptus is too potent to place undiluted on the skin.

- ❀ Blend a few drops with a teaspoon of a mild carrier oil such as almond or sunflower.
- ❀ "Dot" the blend directly on the skin. Make dots along the sinus passages under the cheekbones and up the center of the forehead (see figure #2) for immediate relief.

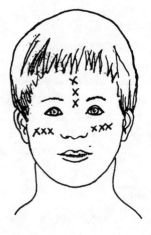

Herbal Snuff

When nothing else is strong enough to break through heavy-duty nasal congestion, Herbal Snuff will do it. This will quickly open and drain the sinuses, and even cause a bout of sneezing. I consider it nothing short of herbal dynamite! Appropriate for the child mature enough to implement the following directions for its inhalation, herbal snuff's ingredients are antimicrobial, antiseptic, and stimulating.

If you do this first, it will encourage your child to try "snuffing." Often, we don't even know we're congested until we try a bit of herbal snuff.

- ❀ Mix together 1 tablespoon each powdered goldenseal root and bayberry bark. Add *just a pinch* of powdered garlic and cayenne.

❀ Place a pencil-point-sized dot of the powdered mixture on the back of your child's hand.

❀ Show your child how to pinch one nostril closed while inhaling the powdered herbs into the other. Repeat on the other side.

❀ Wait about five minutes before allowing your child to blow his nose.

Head-Clearing Tea

During a period of nasal congestion, I find it helpful to make a pot of this decongesting, head-clearing tea to be sipped warm in ½-cup doses throughout the day, as needed.

❀ Combine 1 teaspoon peppermint leaf, ½-teaspoon thyme leaf, and ½-teaspoon sage leaf.

❀ Pour 2 cups boiled water over combined herbs; cover; steep until cool. Add honey to sweeten.

❀ Encourage your child to breathe deeply while slowly sipping the tea.

SWOLLEN GLANDS

One of my clients, five-year-old Caroline, experienced speedy relief from the pain of swollen glands with an old folk remedy, the lymph-clearing carrot-poultice treatment. Once again, your kitchen can be a valuable resource for healing therapies.

Carrot Poultice

❀ Grate a large organic carrot onto a piece of cheesecloth and close it up into a packet.

❀ Hold in place against the swollen gland(s) with your child's favorite scarf or tie and leave in place for as long as is comfortable. In our house, "Bear," a very special stuffed animal, received a matching carrot poultice!

Lymph-Cleansing Tea

The chemical constituents of mullein leaf, echinacea, and red clover blossoms make them excellent lymph/blood cleansers (for swollen glands, mumps, tonsillitis, mononucleosis).

- ❀ Combine 1 teaspoon of each herb, and steep in 2 cups boiled water until cool.
- ❀ Sweeten with honey and give every few hours in ¼- to ½-cup doses, depending upon the size of your child.

The Castor Oil Pack

Edgar Cayce, a 20th century medical intuitive, often recommended castor oil packs for a variety of ailments (see Appendix A). It's ability to mobilize stagnating lymph congestion makes it an ideal remedy for swollen glands. Rather than the traditional, unpleasant tablespoons of castor oil forced internally in days of yore, the castor oil pack is applied externally. This is—as I'm sure your child will agree—a much more pleasant way of administering this wonderful herb.

- ❀ Using cold-pressed castor oil from the health food store, dampen a folded piece of white wool flannel. (There is a packaged flannel designed for castor packs often available at health food stores, or see Appendix G for resources)
- ❀ Apply directly to the swollen gland, covering with a hot water bottle.
- ❀ The pack can be reapplied several times a day for 20 minutes at a time.
- ❀ When you are all finished using the castor oil pack, the residual oil should be cleaned from the skin using a wash of ½ teaspoon baking soda dissolved in ½ cup water. This is to prevent the skin from reabsorbing any toxins the castor oil may have pulled to its surface.

THE COMMON COLD

Herbal Teas

The following herbs bring relief from the congestion, fever, and achiness of a cold:

Elderflower
Peppermint
Yarrow
Boneset
Hyssop
Thyme
Mullein
Echinacea
Sage

- ❀ Prepare an infusion (see Appendix A for directions) by using one or more of the herbs.
- ❀ Give in small, frequent doses (see Chapter 3 for dosing guidelines).
- ❀ If your child is unwilling to drink enough tea, any of the above can be combined to make a bath (see Appendix A for directions), which will allow the herbs to be assimilated into the body via the skin.

Echinacea

- ❀ Dosing according to weight, give liquid echinacea extract, diluted in a little water or juice, every 2 hours until symptoms lessen; then give 3–4 times a day until your child is completely well.
- ❀ Echinacea is a well-respected immune booster, as is vitamin C. Giving a dose of vitamin C (liquid, chewables, or tablets) with every dose of echinacea creates a synergistic response — meaning that when combined, the immune-stimulating action of each substance is enhanced, performing at a higher level.

Garlic

Eat leeks in March and wild garlic in May
And all year after physicians may play.
> —Old Welsh Rhyme

Garlic is well known for its antiviral, antibacterial properties.

- Add a fresh chopped clove of garlic to foods (garlic mashed potatoes, pasta with garlic and oil, and garlic bread are some of my favorites).
- Or, give several drops garlic oil, a garlic tablet, or perle, 3–4 times a day.

Fluids

Hydration is important to the recovery from a cold. In addition to the above teas and water, warm lemonade can be made using fresh lemons, warm water, and honey, to taste.

Inhalations

For the clogged head that accompanies a cold, try one of the suggestions in the section on nasal congestion (page 75).

HERBAL REMEDIES FOR THE MOUTH AND LIPS

Even something as simple as chapped lips can cause a child great discomfort. I tried many over-the-counter oils, jellies, salves, and lipsticks, only to discover (big surprise here!) that herbal formulas worked best.

Castor Oil Lip Salve

There is no simpler therapy for lips than castor oil. I keep it stored in a plastic squeeze bottle next to my bedside and use a drop morning and night on my lips and on the sides of my index fingers. I mention the fingers here as well because it is such a common place for the skin to crack when cold weather arrives.

Herbal Salves and Lipsticks

More often than not, classrooms are overheated and drying to the skin. Children can bring their herbal salves or lipsticks to school and apply them during the day as needed. In cold weather, remind your children to apply salves before going to school or out to play at recess time.

The base of the herbal salve or lipstick is usually beeswax and olive oil—which, by themselves, are soothing, moisturizing, and healing. Look for the addition of aloe, calendula, chamomile, chickweed, comfrey, marshmallow, peppermint, and apply the product preventatively during cold weather or when your child's lips are dry.

Calendula Mouth Rinse

Inflammation of the gums or oral mucosa respond well to a mouth rinse made of calendula's anti-inflammatory and wound-healing properties.

It's fun to make a game of holding the rinse in the mouth. You might sing a nursery rhyme for the allotted time. Any fun distraction will keep the rinse in the mouth longer.

- ✿ Prepare calendula tea by steeping 1 teaspoon of the herb in one cup boiled water.
- ✿ Allow to steep until cooled; strain.
- ✿ Encourage your child to hold a mouthful of the tea on the affected area for up to a minute, 3–4 times a day.
- ✿ The rinse should be spat out after each holding.

COLD SORES

Nutritional Support

Recurrent cold sores (eruptions around the mouth area) indicate the presence of an oral herpes virus. Consult your doctor or nutritionist about giving your child lysine supplements and/or adding lysine-rich foods to the diet. Buckwheat, an easily digested grain, is an excellent food source of lysine. Who could resist a "medicinal" stack of buckwheat pancakes after a cold sore has first made its appearance, or as a nutritional preventative?

Herbal Healers

This would be a good time for your child to benefit from the antiviral, immune-stimulating properties of echinacea as well as garlic (in whatever form your child prefers—perles, oil tablets, raw and chopped on buttered toast).

- Give echinacea and garlic three times a day for the duration of the cold sore, and for a week thereafter.
- The liquid extract of the black walnut, when dabbed on the cold sore several times daily, will dry it up quickly.
- Hold or have your child hold a sliver of raw garlic against the cold sore for 15 to 20 minutes in the morning and before bedtime for the first two days.
- Another effective botanical approach is osha root liquid extract, taken internally (see Chapter 3 for dosing guidelines) as well as applied topically to the cold sore several times a day.

Aloe Leaf Remedy

One of my students uses this remedy on her child and says it prevents the cold sores from erupting, if applied as soon as they are detected. The trick is to keep the aloe leaf from slipping and sliding, and to get it to stay in place overnight when applied to the lip area.

We devised a method that encases the aloe leaf in gauze or cheese-cloth, making it easier to tape into place.

- ✿ When the cold sore first looks or feels like it's going to erupt, cut a piece of aloe leaf (sized to cover the affected area) from the center of a stalk (every home should have an aloe plant available for medicinal use — they're easy to find in plant nurs-eries and so easy to grow).
- ✿ Slit open the leaf to expose the gelatinous inner gel.
- ✿ Encase the piece of aloe in gauze or cheesecloth and apply to the cold sore (with the gel side toward the skin).
- ✿ Tape in place with surgical tape and leave on overnight.

Raspberry Leaf Mouth Rinse

Whether the mouth sores are canker sores, viral sores, or inflamed tissue from braces, a Raspberry Leaf Mouth Rinse will bring relief overnight.

- ✿ Steep 2 tablespoons dried raspberry leaf in 1 cup boiled water until cool.
- ✿ Hold a mouthful of the liquid on the affected area for one minute, 3 times a day; spit out. Be careful not to administer more than 3 times a day, or this rinse will *cause* irritation rather than relieve it.
- ✿ This rinse can be kept in your refrigerator for 3 days.

BLEEDING GUMS

Flossing Can Be Fun

You may think it odd that I'm including a word on bleeding gums in a book for children as this is a problem we usually develop later in life. Moreover, this is one of those health issues that is, for many people, genetically determined. I have friends and clients who take impeccable care of their teeth and still have problems with their gums; other people have never used floss in their life and have super-healthy gums.

Even though bleeding gums usually don't develop until we are in our late teens or twenties, it is important to teach your children early on not only about sugar's negative effects on teeth, but also about why flossing should be a daily practice. Like many things, if children incorporate this into their daily health routine, they'll keep this habit throughout their lives.

While flossing should be done in front of the bathroom mirror at first, it is easy to do by touch after a few weeks of practice. In fact, your kids can floss while watching TV or listening to music. Offer your child flavored floss to keep it fun. As beneficial as flossing is for adults, it is that much more so for kids, as it maintains the gums in the pink of health and can help ensure a lifetime of periodontal health. Ask your dental hygienist to spend time teaching your child how to properly floss the teeth.

Astringent Mouthwash

I suggest making an herbal mouthwash a daily part of your child's health regime as early as possible. Because it is parasites and bacteria that pose the greatest challenge to the health of the gums, a mouthwash of astringent, antimicrobial herbs can help improve their condition in just one week's time. The following liquid extracts may be diluted for this use:

Myrrh
Goldenseal
Echinacea
Oak bark

- ✿ Before each brushing, dilute 5 drops of the equally combined herbs in an ounce of water.
- ✿ Have your child swish around the gums for a minute, then spit out.
- ✿ Brushing afterward will rid the mouth of the herbs' strong taste.

✿ If desired, a drop of oil of peppermint may be added to the formula to improve the taste.

Tea Tree/Peppermint Mouthwash

A less medicinal, more pleasant-tasting antibacterial mouthwash can be made for daily use, or be used as the follow-up to the more astringent mouthwash described above.

✿ Combine 6 drops oil of peppermint with 4 drops tea tree oil in 12 ounces distilled water.

✿ A brief swish around the mouth will leave your child's mouth and breath fresh and minty.

TOOTHACHES

Ouch-tooth! Remedy

My co-writer, David, struck up a conversation with a toddler on the New York City subway (accompanied by his mother, of course). David asked the youngster, "How are you?" "I got a ouch-tooth," the tyke replied. So "ouch-tooth" remedy this is!

Until a painful tooth is treated by your family dentist, you can provide temporary relief, helping both you and your child get through the night. It is the anesthetic properties of these potent essential oils that offer numbing relief.

✿ Add a drop of essential oil of clove or peppermint to a piece of cotton or cotton swab, and hold it on the affected tooth for as long as your child will allow.

✿ This can be reapplied as often as necessary for pain relief.

✿ If possible, wedge the treated cotton between the teeth so that it will stay in place on its own.

The Lower Respiratory System

Parents skeptical about using natural remedies to heal illness are often willing to try a therapy that is applied externally rather than given internally. Lower respiratory issues respond well to topical applications—bronchitis, asthma, coughs, and even pneumonia. (Yes, pneumonia. While antibiotics can help bacterial pneumonia, they can't touch viral pneumonia. Herbs can provide important relief in both cases.)

COUGHS/LARYNGITIS/LUNG CONGESTION

Onion/Honey Cough Syrup

Here's a sweet and delicious cough remedy your child will love to eat! The anti-inflammatory properties of both honey and onion help relax coughing spasms and soothe irritated tissue. Onion and honey are antimicrobial, as well.

Research reveals that onions, as well as garlic and cayenne, produce an irritation in the stomach lining that signals the lungs to release a flow of secretions that help thin sticky, thickened mucus. Can you recall how peeling an onion brings tears to your eyes?

That's the same mechanism in action. This is what makes onion such a good expectorant, breaking up congestion in the lungs.

- ❧ In a small saucepan, mix together 1 cup honey; 1 medium, yellow onion, chopped; 1 teaspoon thyme leaf (more, if you use it fresh).
- ❧ Cook the above ingredients until the onion is softened.
- ❧ Serve warm by itself, eaten by the teaspoonful; over mashed potatoes; or with your child's favorite vegetable, meat, or chicken.
- ❧ Small amounts may be eaten several times a day, if desired.

The healing properties of thyme have often been called upon in another of my passions, directing children's theatre. Sometimes, the fledgling thespians' vocal chords don't hold up for multiple performances, so I share the formula with their parents, suggesting they use it throughout the day. I also recommend that they send their children to the performances with a container of honey-sweetened thyme tea. School plays don't usually have understudies, so you can imagine how important, in the microcosm of the little actors' world, a remedy for laryngitis can be!

Thyme/Honey Syrup

Thyme is an excellent expectorant as well as an antimicrobial herb, and honey not only soothes but is a preservative as well. I keep this wonderful-tasting syrup in my refrigerator all winter long. It can be used for colds, coughs, laryngitis, and sore throats.

- ❧ Steep 1 oz. dried thyme leaf in 1 cup boiled water, covered, until cool.
- ❧ Strain; mix the liquid with 1 cup honey.
- ❧ Store refrigerated in a glass jar. It keeps well for several months.
- ❧ Give undiluted doses of 1 teaspoon to 1 tablespoon several times a day as needed.

Thyme/Eucalyptus Bath

Another way to benefit from the antimicrobial properties of thyme is in an inhalation bath. As thyme is also a bronchodilater, it's a good way to help relieve the constricted breathing that can be experienced with a chest cold, pneumonia, or bronchitis.

Eucalyptus helps stimulate secretions and is antimicrobial. Before immersing your child in this bath, be sure that the eucalyptus is well tolerated. I have found that some allergic, asthmatic children experience just the opposite: a constricted, heavy feeling in the chest.

- Steep 2 tablespoons dried thyme leaf in 1 quart boiled water for 30 minutes; strain; add to bath water.
- Add 4 to 6 drops oil of eucalyptus and stir into bath water.
- Teach your child how to breathe deeply while bathing.

Heavy-Duty Onion Poultice

To break up heavy lung congestion, as in pneumonia, or to soothe the inflammation of bronchitis, consider the anti-inflammatory, antimicrobial, secretion-stimulating action of this treatment. It takes some preparation, but the results are well worth the effort.

- Simmer a large, thinly sliced, yellow onion in water until just softened.
- Place onion on a piece of white cloth (cheesecloth, cotton diaper or linen napkin), and fold up to make a packet.
- Carefully apply to your child's congested area, making sure it is not too hot to the touch, and cover with a terrycloth towel to retain the heat.
- As the onion poultice cools on your child's chest, prepare another one to replace it. This procedure can be repeated several times using fresh onions for each poultice.

The Onion Pack

I've never seen anything work faster to stop incessant coughing than a pack made of yellow onion. When my sons coughed through the night, remaining asleep while I lay awake, I'd head for the kitchen to prepare this remedy. By the time I would get from the bed to the door, the coughing would stop!

The medicinal properties of the onion are contained in its fumes, and the inhalation of them is what does the trick. The room won't smell so fabulous in the morning, but I always figured it was worth a night's sleep.

- ❧ Thinly slice a small yellow onion, place in cheesecloth, folding it over to make a self-contained "pack."
- ❧ Place in a 200-degree oven for just a few minutes to warm it.
- ❧ Place on your child's chest, taping in place with surgical tape and covering with a nightshirt.

Chest-Relaxing Ginger Rub

When your child's chest feels tight as a result of cold or flu and coughing can be painful, a ginger rub will bring herbal heat to the chest. Ginger's stimulating properties increase circulation and help loosen things up. I can remember times when this remedy was so effective that the next night my son required an onion pack to stop the incessant coughing from all the loosened phlegm!

- ❧ To prepare this rub, mix together 1 tablespoon each powdered ginger (purchased from the health food store where it will not have been irradiated) and a non-petrolated petroleum jelly (also available at a health food store).
- ❧ The mixture will look rather like brown frosting. But don't eat it—spread it on your child's chest, then cover with a cotton T-shirt.
- ❧ A reddening of the area is normal and indicates that the ginger

is increasing circulation to the capillaries near the surface of the skin.

❀ In the morning, the petroleum jelly will have been absorbed, and the ginger will have worked its magic, as indicated by your child's ability to breathe more easily.

Another wonderful reason to use ginger: A Brigham Young University study revealed that this herb significantly decreased nausea and diarrhea associated with the 24-hour flu.

Aromatic Congestion Oil

Blending together any of the following essential oils will create a treatment that deeply penetrates tissue, stimulating blood flow to the lung area, helping to open air passages. In addition, the herbs are anti-inflammatory and antimicrobial:

Thyme
Eucalyptus
Peppermint
Lavender
Anise
Cinnamon
Hyssop

❀ For children under eight years of age, blend 4–6 drops combined essential oils in a teaspoon of carrier oil such as almond, apricot kernel, or grapeseed. For the older child, increase the dilution to 10 drops to the teaspoon of oil.

❀ The Congestion Oil may be rubbed on the chest and back in the morning, afternoon, and at bedtime. Cover with a cotton shirt.

❀ Continue treatment until congestion loosens and your child is more comfortable.

❀ You may expect a slight reddening of the skin due to the oils' circulatory-enhancing effect. If your child exhibits more than just a slight reddening or a rash, discontinue use.

❀ Several drops of the Congestion Oil may be used in a bath.
❀ For inhalations, add several drops of the Congestion Oil to a pot of hot water, encouraging your child to breathe deeply over the water.
❀ Several drops of the essential oils may be added to a vaporizer. (Do not mix with carrier oil.)

Echinacea

Echinacea's immune-enhancing properties may be called to action to help the body fight off the respiratory infection. Its chemical properties help to slow the spread of infection while enhancing immune function in the lymphatic system and mucus membranes.

❀ Give oral doses of echinacea every 2 hours (see Chapter 3 for dosing guidelines) until the symptoms diminish, and 3 times a day thereafter until your child is totally well.

For an in-depth discussion of echinacea, see Chapter 12: Immune System Enhancers.

Cold and Flu Tea

Upper and lower respiratory symptoms respond well to the healing properties of the herbs contained in this soothing, decongesting tea. A large quantity of the dried herbs can be mixed and stored in an airtight jar.

4 parts echinacea
2 parts sage leaf
2 parts eucalyptus
1 part ginger root
1 part thyme leaf

How effective is this natural tea? Let's run down the all-star list of the ingredients' properties:

Echinacea stimulates the immune system and is antimicrobial;
Sage leaf detoxifies and decongests;
Eucalyptus leaf decongests and is antimicrobial;
Ginger root detoxifies and stimulates circulation;
Thyme is a decongestant and antimicrobial.

- ❧ Steep 1 teaspoon of the combined herbs in 1 cup boiled water, covered, for 15 minutes. Several cups can be made at one time, warming as needed. Natural honey may be used to sweeten the tea.
- ❧ Initially, an ounce or two may be given every 15 minutes, until relief is experienced, and then ¼ to ½ cup every 2–3 hours.

Garlic: Nature's Antibiotic

My television show, *The Healing Power of Herbs*, contains a segment titled "Uncommon Uses of Common Kitchen Herbs." There is no commonly used herb more potent in its ability to fight respiratory infection than the wondrous garlic bulb.

The next few formulas incorporate garlic for its powerful antiparasitic, antibacterial, antifungal, and antiviral properties. That's a lot of infection-fighting potential for something whose only claim to fame has been as a breath-polluting yet tasty addition to foods!

Known as "Russian penicillin," garlic is valued in that country in its extracted form, which is then vaporized and inhaled. In ancient Egypt, garlic was so highly esteemed that 15 pounds of garlic bulbs bought one slave. In fact, the Egyptians thought garlic so powerful that they placed its cloves in King Tut's tomb to protect him in the great hereafter. I hope you, too, will elevate garlic to "royal" status in your home for the great here and now!

One further word on the magic of garlic: to repel fleas, give fresh or powdered garlic to your family pet.

CMG Syrup

Daytime coughing responds well to the healing properties of comfrey, mullein, and garlic. This combination can be found in Dr.

Christopher's CMG Syrup, or in other formulas in the health food store.

- ✿ Comfrey soothes and helps repair irritated bronchial and lung tissue, and helps the child cough up congesting fluids. (See Appendix H for a special note on comfrey.)
- ✿ Mullein leaf also has an affinity for bronchial and lung tissue and, due to its astringency, helps eliminate excess fluids.
- ✿ Garlic, as discussed above, is widely hailed for its antimicrobial properties. As does cayenne, garlic stimulates the flow of secretions in the stomach which, in turn, signal the lungs to stimulate a flow that helps to thin sticky, thickened mucus, dispersing it for the body to reabsorb. Daily doses of garlic may preventatively keep secretions thinned and flowing.
- ✿ Give ½ to 1 teaspoon of the syrup, diluted in an ounce of water or juice, 3–4 times a day.

Garlic Fever Reducer

To bring down a high fever, especially when associated with bronchial congestion:

- ✿ Put enough fresh cloves of garlic in a blender to make a paste that will spread ¼" thick on gauze.
- ✿ Lightly coat the soles of your child's feet with olive oil so the garlic does not irritate them.
- ✿ Affix the garlic gauze pads to the soles of the feet with roller gauze; cover with cotton socks.
- ✿ Leave on overnight, provide plenty of water to drink, and watch the fever go down.
- ✿ If necessary, more garlic paste may be applied as it is absorbed by the body.

By the way, garlic is so powerfully absorbed through the soles of the feet that, in short time, your child will have garlic breath!

Dr. Christopher's Anti-Plague Syrup

While its name sounds rather intimidating, it indicates this formula's effectiveness for all kinds of infections. Consisting of fresh garlic juice, apple cider vinegar, and other potent antimicrobial herbs, it is an excellent therapy for active respiratory infection. This syrup is also an excellent post-infection support for the body as it recuperates.

- ❀ From infancy to age 4, give ⅛–¼ teaspoon 3 or 4 times a day.
- ❀ Ages 5–10 should receive ¼–½ teaspoon.
- ❀ Ages 10 and older, ½–1 teaspoon.
- ❀ This syrup has a strong taste and is more palatable diluted in a bit of juice.

Lung Formula Tea

This formula gently expels matter from the lungs and bronchials, and is excellent for a more intense cough, as well as for asthma. It contains equal parts dried comfrey (a soothing expectorant), mullein and sage (antimicrobial and expectorant), and chickweed (soothing and anti-inflammatory).

- ❀ In an acute situation, when coughing is intense and persistent, you can give droppersful of it to your child every 15–30 minutes until relief is attained.
- ❀ As a tonic, give ¼ cup 3 or 4 times a day to expel matter from the lungs and bronchials. Continue until the chest sounds clear.

Fluids

The best and most important fluid for the body is good quality water. At all times, but especially during periods of illness, the body's need for water must be met to enable the proper manufacturing of proteins, enzymes, and hormones. When the body is physically compromised, it must be kept well hydrated so that its chemical processes facilitate healing and the flushing of toxins—and this is especially true for infants and children.

Cell Salts

For a description and dosing guidelines see Appendix F. *The Biochemic Handbook* provides the following suggestions for coughs.

> *Ferr. Phos.* for hard, dry cough with soreness and fever.
>
> *Kali Mur.* for cough with white, albuminous phlegm; white- or gray-coated tongue, children's cough.
>
> *Kali Sulph.* for cough with yellow expectoration, which becomes worse in a heated room or in the evening.
>
> *Mag. Phos.* for painful, spasmodic cough with a tendency to persist.
>
> *Calc. Sulph.* for a cough that is loose and rattling, with expectoration of thin, watery sputum. To be given in alteration with Ferr. Phos.
>
> *Silica* for cough accompanied by thick, yellow-green, profuse expectoration.
>
> *Calc. Phos.* is useful as an intercurrent remedy and during convalescence.

The Biochemic Handbook provides the following remedies for symptoms of bronchitis, some of which seem appropriate to give at the first sign of a cold with the intention of preventing further involvement.

> *Ferr. Phos.* at early signs of inflammation and temperature.
>
> *Kali Sulph.* to be alternated with Ferr. Phos. to promote perspiration and control fever. (Continue this cell salt if expectoration is yellow and slimy, and for evening aggravation of symptoms.)
>
> *Kali Mur.* at the second stage, when a feeling of stuffiness and whitish-gray tongue is accompanied by thick, white phlegm.

Nat. Mur. for watery, frothy expectoration with concomitant loss
   of taste and smell.
Calc. Sulph. a useful remedy to be given in alternation with
   Calc. Phos. to speed recovery during your child's
   convalescence.

Suggested Protocol

In addition, the following are suggested protocols for children with
colds who are prone to lower respiratory illness.

- Provide echinacea every 2 hours (see Chapter 3 for dosing
  guidelines).
- Keep the body thoroughly hydrated with good quality water by
  offering frequent sips.
- Provide fresh garlic, oil of garlic, or garlic tablets, 3 times a
  day.
- Avoid dairy foods, which are mucus-forming. (Your child does
  not need the additional burden of more mucus at this time.)
- Be certain that your child's bowels are moving easily each day,
  since constipation and the consequent retention of toxins puts
  additional burden on the chest area.
- Give acidophilus tablets or liquid 3 to 4 times a day. (See p.
  210 for further description.)

At the first sign of chest involvement, add to the above:

- Lung Formula Tea
- Appropriate cell salts
- Additional herbal therapies as needed

ASTHMA

For some children, asthma can be quite a simple issue to resolve;
for others, it can be life threatening. The same toxins that cause

eczema in one child, or sinus congestion in another, can cause the breathing tubes to constrict in a genetically predisposed child. Skin and sinus issues are uncomfortable, but a fight for breath can be terrifying.

There are many natural ways to approach asthma. Hopefully, by implementing them you can keep your child's condition under control. If the asthma requires medication, perhaps you can keep it to a minimum by combining it with natural approaches.

As I see it, in addition to genetics, there are five basic challenges to the child with asthma:

1. Environmental toxins
2. Food intolerance
3. Emotional stress
4. Physical exertion (as in sports)
5. Infection

You may not be able to alter the genetic patterns that have set your child up to express toxins in the lower respiratory area, but you can take charge of your child's exposure to those toxins, thereby minimizing the challenges and discomfort.

Environmental Toxins

Because humans are such diverse beings, there is no official checklist telling us which pollutants will cause your child's airways to contract. Below is a list you should be aware of, noting your child's reaction when in the presence of each. The tricky thing is that exposure to one toxin may not set your child off, but when it is in addition to the presence of another toxin, it might. Keeping a diary helps, as does keen observation.

- Recirculated air found in malls, airplanes, and office buildings
- Unclean filters used in home or office air conditioners, air purifiers, and heating systems
- Pollen and mold spores

- ✿ High ozone counts, "bad air" days, smog, factory air pollution
- ✿ Cleaning products (home, office, and laundry). Restaurants often allow staff to clean floors and tabletops while you are dining—watch out!
- ✿ Chemicals in newly purchased, unlaundered clothing and linens
- ✿ Dust in the home (Check curtains, carpeting, stuffed animals—behind, above, and below everything.)
- ✿ Fragrances (perfume, perfumed samples in magazines, fragranced products)
- ✿ Classroom threats (including paint, chalk, newspaper ink, naptime bedding, and marking pens)
- ✿ Exhaust fumes from autos and machinery
- ✿ Chlorine in swimming pools and cleaning products
- ✿ Damp, musty places, bedding and clothing
- ✿ Houseplant mold
- ✿ Outdoor barbecue fumes
- ✿ Essential oils
- ✿ Fireplaces
- ✿ Beauty salon chemicals
- ✿ Cigarette/cigar/pipe smoke
- ✿ Animal dander and feathers, feather pillows, down comforters and jackets

If this makes you want to put your youngster in a padded cell, then at least be sure the padding has been washed in natural detergent!

- ✿ In addition to aggressively keeping your home free of environmental toxins, an air purifier/ionizer can significantly help to cleanse the air of fungus, bacteria, and chemical odors. I use them throughout my home and office, and have found the air quality to be noticeably improved, even refreshing. See Appendix G for information on this subject.

For many children, an accumulation of toxins is what sets them off.

❀ So if it's your child's allergy season, be more careful about what additional toxins the body is experiencing.

❀ Perhaps certain foods should be avoided during pollen season so that your child can better tolerate the practically unavoidable exposure to airborne pollens.

In her book, *Encyclopedia of Natural Healing for Children and Infants* (Keats, 1996), Dr. Mary Bove recommends giving your child magnesium and vitamin C before physical exertion to help prevent an asthmatic attack. Magnesium relaxes smooth muscles, and vitamin C helps stabilize chemicals that may act as triggers. Consult a nutritionist for doses appropriate to your child.

In my radio show, "Revealing Secrets for Mind and Body," I had the pleasure of interviewing Dr. Bill Wolverton about his book, *How to Grow Fresh Air: 50 Houseplants that Purify Your Home or Office* (Penguin, 1997). Dr. Wolverton is a retired NASA research scientist and one of the world's foremost authorities in the use of natural processes for environmental pollution control. His photographs and simple charts make it easy to select the best houseplants to purify your environment; many of these plants are easily found in any greenhouse or plant store. Plants are not just visual treats but nature's living air purifiers!

Comparing nature with the human body, Dr. Wolverton explains:

❀ The rain forest acts as the earth's lungs, producing oxygen and removing carbon dioxide.

❀ Human lungs breathe in the plants' oxygen and exhale carbon dioxide.

❀ The wetlands function as the earth's kidneys, with the aquatic plants filtering nutrients and environmental toxins from the water as it flows back into streams, rivers, and oceans.

❀ Our kidneys filter impurities from our bloodstream.

An interesting fact to be noted for children with mold sensitivity: plant-filled rooms contain 50–60% fewer airborne molds and bacteria than rooms without plants. Dr. Wolverton has developed fan-assisted planters that can be as effective as 200 plants in removing toxins from one's personal breathing zone. You can obtain a catalogue from Wolverton Environmental Services (601-798-5875).

Food Intolerance

The vagus nerve feeds both the stomach and the bronchial tubes. An offending food can irritate the vagus nerve; this, in turn, causes increased mucus secretions and constriction in the muscular rings that surround the bronchial tubes.

A sensitivity to certain foods may or may not be the root cause of your child's asthma, but it can certainly exacerbate this condition. Dairy is the number one food to be avoided since it is a mucus-producing and mucus-thickening food, and the asthmatic child is already challenged by an excess of thickened mucus.

The younger child's diet is pretty much under your control. You can take charge! You can't change genetic patterns, but you can influence food intake. I've given you a wonderful tool in Appendix C for testing foods; it's called kinesiology, or muscle testing. You can use it to ascertain which foods your child is sensitive to, then eliminate them from the diet. If you're not comfortable testing the foods yourself, then bring your child and the foods you suspect to a health practitioner who includes kinesiology in his or her practice, and let them do the tests for you.

If you can successfully eliminate the poorly tolerated foods from your child's diet, you can remove some of the burden from the immune system. It can then work more effectively to resist other challenging substances in the child's environment.

- ✿ Beware of food additives, especially sulfites and MSG. Monosodium glutamate can be hidden in food products under the label "hydrolyzed protein" and "flavorings."
- ✿ Sulfites are often found in dried fruits. Look for "unsulfured" dried fruits in the health food store. Commercially prepared salads usually contain sulfites, as can grocery store herbs.

As the parent of a child with asthma, you must be more diligent than other parents about checking the sources of the food you and your child eat.

Empower Your Child!

Of course, school-aged children can (and will) get their hands on forbidden foods all too easily.

- ❧ Help your child to understand the consequences of eating the wrong foods.
- ❧ Understanding develops empowerment and responsibility. It also helps develop self-esteem and diminishes that helpless feeling of being a victim of one's own body's fragile airways—especially when the other kids don't have the same problem to deal with.

It's also important for you to recognize that food sensitivities can change over time.

- ❧ Assure your child you will test the offending foods at some point in the future, and will reintroduce them into the diet if they are well tolerated.
- ❧ Explaining to your child that eating these foods will make him feel worse because of the environmental problems in the classroom may help him to resist food temptations.
- ❧ Similarly, it is important that you alert the child's teachers to potential classroom hazards so that they are aware of the problem.
- ❧ Be sure to provide the foods that are safe for your child, and those that promote general health.
- ❧ Make them taste good and look appetizing. (Remember, they're in direct competition with those colorful and "tasty" foods that are absolutely laden with chemicals and dyes.) In fact, if they're interesting enough, other children will want to sample your kids' goodies—and imagine how delighted your child will be to share his food with friends.

❀ But be sure to caution your child against food swaps. One doesn't have to receive to give!

While we're on the subject of food, I'd like to share with you a nugget of wisdom from Dr. John R. Christopher. Decades ago, Dr. Christopher advocated "eating from under your own fig tree," which meant that food was healthiest for you when eaten in season from your own locale. This advice presciently predates the dangerous agricultural chemicals now used to grow our foods. Chemicals considered too harmful to pass U.S. standards are often shipped to other countries, used on their produce, and then exported back to America. Ironically, we pay a premium for imported foods containing chemicals considered too harmful for our own farmers to use!

To Restore Emotional Balance

Empower your child with the ability to bring the emotions back into check. The following techniques require your help and input at first, but once your child understands how to use them, she can do it on her own.

❀ Visualizations can be created to help your child imagine the airways opening. This is a very effective tool, one used by corporate executives, sports figures, and cancer patients. Many books have been written about the subject, and with each new day, conventional medical practitioners are adding this therapy to health programs they prescribe. If you prefer, an expert in the field can help design the imagery. (See Appendix E on healing imagery for further details.)

❀ Meditation techniques relax the body and mind. Anyone, at any age, can meditate anywhere. Seek professional guidance in this area or read one of the many books written about meditation. There are even books written about meditation for children.

❀ Focused breathwork is a technique that can strengthen the lungs and teach your child how to breathe more effectively.

You can discuss this approach with a practitioner who is trained in this area.

⚘ Bach Flower Essences can help your child deal with ongoing emotional challenges. A special formula can be created for your child's emotional needs. See Appendix I on Bach Flower Essences for further information on this versatile family of homeopathic remedies.

⚘ Nervine herbs can be used to help a child through a period of emotional stress. Valerian, passionflower, lemon balm, and hops are classic nervine herbs that nourish and calm the nervous system.

Physical Exertion/Adrenal Nourishment

Many children experience exercise-induced asthma when playing sports or other physically challenging activities. The stress-sensitive adrenal glands, when depleted, can cause a drain on the bronchials, inducing wheezing.

⚘ Licorice root helps rid the bronchials of excess mucus by supplying a natural form of cortisone, an anti-inflammatory substance, and also feeds the adrenal glands.

⚘ Give a dose of the liquid extract of licorice root just before your child heads off to sports or any physical activity. Halftime in a football game or time-outs in soccer are great opportunities to provide a second dose, if needed. See Chapter 3 for dosing guidelines.

⚘ Sugar depletes the adrenals. Be sure your child has eaten a healthy meal before engaging in strenuous physical activity.

⚘ Check your health food store for herbal formulations and homeopathics designed to support the adrenals.

⚘ Be sure your child is well hydrated before and during physical activity. Bottled or filtered water is always preferable.

⚘ A torque here, a twist there; before you know it, a subluxation of the spine, a vertebrae out of place. Chiropractic adjustments can have a beneficial effect on adrenal function, as well as strengthen the lung area.

Infection

When a child with asthma gets a cold, you can usually count on it moving into the chest. This, inevitably, is followed by coughing, wheezing—and the cycle begins again. Check out the herbal protocols for cold and flu prevention because, in preventing a cold, you've effectively prevented another asthma attack.

If a respiratory infection has already set in, refer to the chapters on herbal therapies for the upper and lower respiratory systems. If your child's immune system is low in energy, it will impact the weaker parts of the body. To be sure energy is not being drawn from the bronchial/lung area, keep the immune system as strong as possible. (See the Chapter 12 on immune-enhancing herbs for further reference and preventative herbal treatments.)

Herbal Therapies for Asthmatic Attacks

- ❧ Cayenne's circulatory-stimulating and broncho-dilating properties make it an excellent strengthener of the lungs and bronchials. The same way hot cayenne pepper in food can make your eyes water is how it causes a flow of secretions in the bronchial passages, thinning the mucus so it can be dispersed and reabsorbed by the body. It can be given on an ongoing basis, 3 times a day, as a long-term therapy. If your child is having an asthma attack, you can dose cayenne every 10 minutes. You must be the judge of whether your child can deal with the burning sensation cayenne causes to the throat area. (See Chapter 3 for how to administer cayenne.)
- ❧ Valerian, blue cohosh, and lobelia are excellent antispasmodic herbs. Use liquid extracts of these herbs, in combination, to help your child during an attack. Based on an adult dose of about 40 drops of the combined herbs, dose your child according to weight (see Chapter 3 for dosing guidelines). Start with

equal parts valerian and blue cohosh, then add *just a few drops* of lobelia, a powerful antispasmodic. (*Important:* be careful not to overdose lobelia, which could cause vomiting. But do not be afraid of the proper dosage because it acts as a catalyst to the other herbs.) A dose of this combined herbal preparation, diluted in a little water or juice, can be given every 15 minutes during an asthma attack.

❧ Breathe Easy tea by Traditional Medicinals contains herbs that help stop wheezing. To prepare, steep the tea bag for 15–20 minutes, covered, in a cup of boiled water.

❧ Dr. Christopher's Resp-Free formula, available in capsules or liquid, helps clear the lung area of mucus, is antispasmodic, and anti-inflammatory. It is an excellent formula for ongoing therapy and specific asthma attacks. (See Appendix G for resources and Appendix H for ingredients.)

❧ Hot lemonade helps thin mucus and relaxes spasms. Prepare this to taste with freshly squeezed lemons (not commercially prepared lemon juice!), hot water, and honey.

❧ Homeopathic remedies specifically designed for your child's constitution can be helpful in alleviating asthma. Consult a homeopathic physician for best results. (See Appendix G for locating a homeopathic physician in your area.)

❧ Cell salts provide excellent relief from asthma. *The Biochemic Handbook* (see Appendix F for further description of these homeopathic remedies) lists the following cell salts for asthma, depending upon symptoms:

Kali Phos. Nervous asthma, hay asthma. The chief remedy for the breathing and depressed nervous state.

Mag. Phos. Spasmodic nervous asthma. In alternation with Kali Phos.

Kali Mur. With gastric derangement, tongue coated white and mucus white.

Nat. Mur. Profuse, frothy mucus and tears streaming when coughing.

Calc. Phos. Bronchial asthma, clear, tough, gluey expectoration.

Kali Sulph. Bronchial asthma with yellow expectoration. Worse in the evening or in a hot, stuffy atmosphere.

Nat. Sulph. Asthma due to humid conditions with greenish, copious expectoration.

At the very least, these descriptions will make you take a closer look at your child's symptoms. And, if used as recommended, cell salts really can help bring asthma under control.

Honegar

⚘ Honegar (apple cider vinegar and honey) helps restore pH (acid/alkaline balance) in the body, which can be helpful in stopping wheezing. Combine a tablespoon of apple cider vinegar with a teaspoon of honey and mix with ½ cup warm water. Allow your child to sip this mixture when in distress.

Pressure Points

⚘ Acupressure can also help. There are acupressure points along the spine in the thoracic (lung) area that can help stop wheezing. Use your thumbs to hold these points for as long as your child will allow. These points will probably be sensitive at first, but if held long enough can bring enough energy to the bronchials to relax them and provide much-needed relief. (See figure #3.)

The Integrated Approach

Please understand that the natural approach to asthma does not mean immediately withdrawing your child's medication. Instead, introduce these natural therapies concurrent with asthmatic drugs. As these therapies strengthen the bronchial/lung area, less of the medication may be required and, with the guidance of your pediatrician, can be slowly tapered off, replaced by the safe, natural supports discussed here. Eventually, by further strengthening the lungs

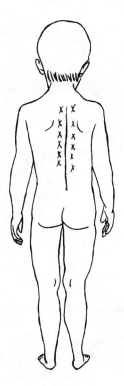

and immune system, and by eliminating poorly tolerated foods, managing environmental issues, and helping your child better cope with stress, you may even be able to withdraw the natural supports.

You may find the natural approach to asthma management a bit overwhelming at first. That's understandable, since North Americans are accustomed to the "silver bullet" approach; that is, let a magic pill do all the work. Take it one step at a time, make changes gradually, and you will find encouragement in the positive response from your child—and, more importantly, from the relief your child feels.

7

Skin-Loving Herbs

How Herbs Penetrate the Skin

The skin's ability to absorb essential oils, herbs, or any other substance is often unappreciated. Essential oils penetrate right into the deep layers of the skin; from there, they can travel to various organs, glands, and tissues of the body. Once essential oils have passed through the epidermis, they seep into the small capillaries in the dermis, and are carried throughout the body by the bloodstream. They are also taken up by the lymph fluid that bathes every cell in the body.

A simple test you can carry out yourself shows just how effectively herbs can be absorbed by and transported around the body. Rub the soles of your child's feet with a clove of garlic. A few hours later, you will be able to smell garlic on your child's breath!

The search for the special formula that will produce great-looking skin is an ageless pursuit. Herbs are potent players in the clearing of adolescent breakouts as well as nourishment for aging skin. Botanicals are also powerful healers of a wide range of skin discomforts, from poison ivy to eczema to insect bites.

The Simple Pimple Fix

I remember the very first time I used a banana to clear Brian's adolescent pimples. He so very much wanted his skin to be clear for the next day's school photographs, and was hoping I had a quick fix. His breakouts looked like they contained material that needed drawing out. Remembering how well banana drew out things like splinters from the skin, we decided to give it a try. I smeared the pulp of a ripened, mashed banana all over his face (the very same remedy I used to give him when he was a baby and had diarrhea!), then let it dry before he went to bed. I don't know which one of us was more overjoyed at the morning's results, but it sure did the trick. His skin was smooth and clear and, by his standards, qualified as photographable.

HIVES

Hives represent an allergic reaction to a substance the body is viewing as a foreign invader. They may look like raised welts or mosquito bites and itch a lot. Recurrent or chronic cases of hives need a little detective work to determine the cause. Often hives are the result of offending foods or a topical product (soap, fragrance, or cosmetic) to which your child is sensitive. Hives can also be a response to the by-product of stress hormones; in other words, anxiety can cause hives in some children. If your child suddenly develops hives for no apparent reason, the first thing to check for is a drug reaction.

Nature's Pharmacy

While you are playing detective, nature's pharmacy could be working to relieve the symptoms and calm your child. Any of the following anti-inflammatory remedies may provide relief from itching. (For directions on specific preparations, see Appendix A on preparing herbal remedies.)

- chamomile compress
- vitamin E oil
- chickweed bath/ointment/compress
- ointment containing soothing herbs like comfrey, calendula, marshmallow root, and/or chickweed
- paste of baking soda, moistened with chamomile tea
- slice of onion
- Dr. Christopher's BF&C ointment (See Appendix H for ingredients and Appendix G for resources.)
- Nat. Mur. cell salt (available in health food stores; see Appendix F for discussion of cell salts.)
- Oatmeal bath (Add a couple of handsful to the bath water.)
- Catnip (Make a quart of the infusion and add to bath water.)

If your child's hives are emotionally based, add:

- Chamomile tea or Tranquili-Tea (See section on Herbs to Calm the Nervous System in Chapter 11.)
- Rescue Remedy, given both topically and internally (See Appendix I on Bach Flower Essences.)

INSECT BITES/STINGS

See Chapter 4, Herbs to the Rescue, for herbal remedies that relieve itch, inflammation, and pain.

HEAD LICE

It is not at all uncommon for preschool and young elementary-aged children to suffer from head lice. Every fall I receive an onslaught of calls from distressed parents whose children suffer from this condition. Typically, the shampoos most doctors prescribe have not been very effective; and, given the harsh chemicals that are being absorbed into the child's scalp, many parents prefer to use a natural approach. Referring to the beginning of this chapter, keep in mind that chemicals used on the skin are absorbed into the bloodstream.

Preventive Measures

- ❀ To help prevent the spread of head lice, obvious hygienic measures should be taught in advance of the first day of school. Teach your child not to wear another child's hat, not to lie on someone else's blanket, not to swap barrettes, other hair accessories, etc.
- ❀ The healthier your child is, the more resistant she will be to parasitic attacks; thus, her diet should be free of sugar, white flour, and junk food to the fullest extent possible. Forgive the comparison, but it is well known that dogs with the healthiest diets are more resistant to fleas. (In fact, if you feed your dog and cat garlic, they will almost always be flea-free!)
- ❀ If dealing with a lice infestation or, if you know of one going around your child's school, to help prevent one, be sure to wash your child's clothes, linens, combs, and brushes in hot water with the addition of a little bit of bleach.

Rosemary Hair Juice

If you are aware of a head-lice epidemic, you can spray your child's head with a preventative, antiparasitic treatment of rosemary tea each morning before she goes off to school.

- ❀ Simmer 4 teaspoons rosemary in 3 cups water for 15 minutes.
- ❀ Turn off the heat, cover, and let sit until cool.
- ❀ Strain and pour into a spray bottle. This infusion can be kept in the refrigerator for 3 days.

Anise Lice Be-Gone

If, despite your best preventative efforts, your child has an itchy head, check for gray lumps, which are lice. If you see colorless dots along strands of the hair, these are nits, the lices' eggs.

This combination of antimicrobial essential oils and olive oil helps to interfere with the lice's cellular metabolism, causing them to smother and die.

- ❦ If you do detect head lice or eggs, combine one teaspoon (one tablespoon for very long, thick, or coarse hair) anise seed oil with 2 teaspoons (2 tablespoons for long, thick, or coarse hair) olive oil, and rub into your child's scalp and hair.
- ❦ Remove lice and eggs by combing through the hair using a metal lice comb. (Your pet's flea comb will also work well.)
- ❦ Repeat this process twice daily until your child is completely free of all infestation.

Tea Tree Oil

Tea tree oil can be used as a comb-through in place of the anise seed/olive oil combination.

- ❦ Add 15 drops tea tree oil to a cup of water.
- ❦ Rub into your child's scalp and hair, then comb through with a metal lice comb, making sure to remove as much matter as possible.

Overnight Lice Treatment

The following combination of antiparasitic essential oils can be used as an overnight treatment to kill off the lice.

2 teaspoons tea tree
2 teaspoons eucalyptus
½ teaspoon rosemary
½ teaspoon lavender

- ❦ Combine essential oils with ½ cup olive oil and apply generously to hair and scalp.
- ❦ Cover your child's head with a shower cap and protect the bed linens with a towel.

❀ Comb through in the morning.

❀ Repeat this treatment nightly until all signs of lice and nits have disappeared.

❀ Repeat twice weekly until the problem has subsided, and the lice "epidemic" is over in school.

❀ After the oil comb-through, you can follow up with a shampoo made with tea tree oil, or add a few drops tea tree oil to her shampoo. The oil of the Australian tea tree is an effective antiparasitical treatment.

Garlic and Echinacea

❀ Give your child a dose of garlic 2–3 times a day (a fresh clove chopped into food, several drops oil of garlic in food or juice, or garlic tablets) for its antiparasitic properties.

❀ This would be a good time to put your child on a 10-day round of echinacea. Give her this herb 3 times a day to stimulate her immune system and help prevent infection that could arise as a result of scratching. (Swollen glands are a sign that infection has developed.) See Chapter 5 for more information on treatment of swollen glands.

RASHES

As is the case with hives, you want to find the etiology of the rash so that it doesn't reoccur. If the rash is itchy, try any of the remedies recommended under Hives, above. If your child's skin is inflamed, but there is no accompanying itch, try:

Soothing Applications

❀ Castor oil, applied topically

❀ Chamomile compress

❀ Dr. Christopher's BF&C ointment

    ❀ Comfrey ointment
    ❀ Plain, organic yogurt, applied topically

Dry It Up

If your child's rash is oozing, the quickest remedy to dry it up is one you can purchase in any pharmacy: Domeboro, a boric acid solution.

    ❀ Dissolve the powder in warm water according to package directions.
    ❀ Immerse a soft cloth, and compress the rash for 20 minutes, 3 times a day.

CHICKEN POX

Skin Relief

Dr. Christopher's BF&C ointment is the all-time winning formula for the itch of chicken pox.

    ❀ Playing "find the spot, ditch the itch," especially with younger children, I like to give them the pot of ointment (supervised, of course, and where age-appropriate), so they can apply it themselves. You'll be amazed to see how quickly their discomfort is relieved when your children help heal themselves! Here, BF&C (which actually stands for bone, flesh, & cartilage) means "Best for Chicken Pox."

Sores in the mouth or throat may be relieved with a rinse/gargle made of a cooled infusion of raspberry leaf. See section on Herbal Remedies for Mouth and Lips on page 80 for formula and dosing.

    ❀ To prevent scarring, apply comfrey ointment, castor oil, or vitamin E oil to areas where scabs have fallen off.
    ❀ "Scarmassage," lotion or ointment, recommended by 20th cen-

tury medical intuitive Edgar Cayce, contains olive oil, peanut oil, camphor, and lanolin. These ingredients, as do those mentioned above, keep the skin moisturized and promote circulation, encouraging the growth of healthy new skin. I suggest applying just a spot of "Scarmassage" on a nonchallenged area at first, to test whether your child is sensitive to any of the ingredients. Lanolin may cause problems in someone sensitive to wool; peanut oil must be avoided by the child allergic to peanuts. "Scarmassage" is available through Heritage Products (800-726-2232).

Support the Immune System

- ✿ Echinacea helps support the immune system while dealing with the virus of chicken pox. (See Chapter 12.)
- ✿ For herbal remedies for fever see page 158.

INFECTED SKIN

There are several highly effective botanical approaches to treating a cut or wound that has become infected.

Sage Wash

- ✿ Steep 2 teaspoons antimicrobial, astringent sage leaf in 1 cup boiled water until cooled.
- ✿ Pour ¼ cup of the tea over the infected area several times a day.
- ✿ Allow to air dry or gently pat dry before covering with a bandage and, if needed, an herbal treatment (see sections on cuts and wounds in Chapter 4).
- ✿ Do not reuse the tea that has been poured over the skin.

Tea Tree Oil

- ✿ Dilute several drops antimicrobial, antiseptic tea tree oil in 1 cup cool water.

- Pour ¼ cup of the liquid over the infected area several times a day.
- Allow to air dry or gently pat dry before covering with a bandage and, if needed, an herbal treatment (see sections on cuts and wounds in Chapter 4).
- Do not reuse the tea that has been poured over the skin.

Note: To benefit from the antiseptic herbs' action throughout the day and night:

- Saturate gauze with one of the above washes.
- Affix to the infected area with surgical tape, and cover with plastic to keep moist.
- During the day, renew with a fresh application every 3 to 4 hours.

Echinacea Paste

Echinacea, in its dried and powdered form, may be mixed with a little water to make a paste, and then applied to the infected area.

- Mix enough powdered herb and water to thoroughly cover the infected tissue.
- Cover with gauze and surgical tape.
- Refresh 4 times a day by adding more of the paste to what is already there.

Echinacea is a powerful blood cleanser; it is this property that cleanses infection from a wound. My son, Brian, tried to break a terrible fall from his bike with the palm of his hand, causing gravel to embed in the skin, resulting in a serious infection. The hand surgeon we consulted said "a procedure" would be required to remove the gravel if Brian's body did not reject it on its own.

With the spectre of this "procedure" (one of my least favorite medical euphemisms) looming large, I proceeded to aggressively treat Brian's hand several times a day, and watched closely to see if the gravel was being rejected. It was not. With just a few days remaining until the next doctor's visit, I tried a new approach. First, I covered my son's palm overnight with a ripened banana peel. Since I knew of banana's ability to remove splinters, I hoped its drawing action would work to pull out the gravel . . . and it did! Next, I put powdered echinacea to work, as described above; it cleansed the wound beautifully and restored a healthy pink tone to Brian's previously gray, infected hand.

So potent is echinacea's blood cleansing action that I have even used it according to its historical Native American use: to cleanse the venom of a snake bite. (See the section on echinacea in Chapter 12 for more on this.)

WARTS

Once again, the oil of the castor bean plant contributes its amazing properties to the healing of our bodies. My first experience of castor oil was with my five-year-old's warts. One or two on the sole of each foot quickly multiplied into ten, prompting me to research Edgar Cayce's remedy for wart removal using castor oil. I followed Cayce's directions carefully, which included stopping the treatment after three weeks of nightly applications (even though the warts were still quite evident). I must admit I thought the therapy was a failure at that point. Much to my surprise, within the following week all the warts dried up, turned black, and fell off, never to return. Now that's a successful treatment!

The Castor Oil Wart Chaser

The combination of the vibrational properties of the castor oil and the pH balancing of the baking soda help to create an inhospitable environment for the wart.

- ✿ In the palm of your hand, add just enough castor oil to ¼ teaspoon baking soda to make a paste. Cover the wart with the paste, keeping it in place with surgical tape. Leave on overnight, removing the tape in the morning.

✿ Repeat nightly for three weeks and then stop . . . and watch the magic happen.

If the wart has been on your child's body for a long time, it may require a second three-week treatment, but wait a couple of weeks before resuming the nightly applications. If, initially, there is irritation, it is from the baking soda and you can expect this to disappear soon.

ECZEMA AND CHRONIC RASHES

Eczema is an allergic response, often to a food, detergent, fabric, bubble bath, or other irritant. Playing detective can help you locate the source of the problem, which can then be eliminated from your child's environment. (See more about how to be a great natural healing detective in the section on allergies in Chapter 12.)

Chickweed

Chickweed's anti-inflammatory properties make it extremely soothing and healing to eczematous skin. This excellent herb for clearing eczema can be found in health food stores in the form of an ointment (usually in a base of olive oil and beeswax), and as a dried herb, which can be prepared as a bath. The ointment is, of course, more convenient, and can be reapplied several times a day, but can also be used after a chickweed bath for longer-lasting protection.

Chickweed Bath

The bath is a soothing way to prepare your child for bed.

✿ Steep 8 tablespoons dried chickweed herb in 2 quarts boiled water for 30 minutes.

✿ Strain and add to bath water. Have your child soak in the bath for 20 minutes.

✿ Another way to prepare a chickweed bath is by filling a muslin pouch or a washcloth tied with a rubber band with the dried chickweed herb, and hanging it from the faucet as the water fills the tub.

✿ For a weepy rash, I recommend adding a 2-cup infusion of calendula flowers or one cup apple cider vinegar (for their antiseptic properties) to your child's chickweed bath.

✿ Individual areas may be treated with compresses of calendula or apple cider vinegar.

Inner Cleansing

With skin rashes of any kind, it is often the case that cleansing what you can't see brings healing to the part of the body you can see. Herbs that cleanse the liver and bloodstream help to clear the skin. You can give diluted extracts or teas 3 times a day. I find it most interesting that the parts of herbs that reach deepest into the earth— their roots—are also the parts that reach deepest into our bodies to cleanse them. Look for a combination of cleansing herbs:

Yellow dock root
Burdock root
Dandelion root
Sarsaparilla root
Barberry root
Oregon grape root

Itchy-Skin Reliever

Skin that itches—as a result of insect bites, rashes, etc.—often responds well to slices of potato applied directly to the skin. White or red potato is best; this vegetable is also a well-known folk remedy for relieving joint pain. Its medicinal value is in its low content of alkaloids and their ability to neutralize acidity.

- ❀ Thinly slice potato and affix to skin with surgical tape.
- ❀ Cover with plastic, if desired.
- ❀ Leave in place for several hours or overnight.

PRICKLY HEAT RASH

An occasional appearance of prickly heat rash can be soothed with:

- ❀ Aloe gel applied directly to rash; cover with gauze, if desired.
- ❀ Slippery elm bark powder thickly applied to affected area; cover with gauze, if desired.
- ❀ Baths of chamomile, calendula, or chickweed provide soothing soaks for irritated skin.

A chronic case of prickly heat indicates the need to cool down your child's internal, as well as external, body.

- ❀ Excess internal heat is often caused by poorly digested foods. See Appendix C for how to test for food sensitivities.
- ❀ Be sure your child is having daily, easy bowel movements. Congested bowels also heat up the body. See page 247, and 249 for bowel-cleansing herbs.
- ❀ Acidophilus helps to restore intestinal balance benefiting the skin. See pages 210 and 211 for how to use.
- ❀ Cooling teas of chamomile, nettles, or peppermint may also help. Give three times a day until the rash clears up.

CYSTS

I have seen many instances where a cyst on the surface of the skin looked like it would need surgical removal but . . .

Magical Castor Oil

- ✿ Instead, magical castor oil, applied 2 to 3 times a day to the affected area for 3 weeks' time, did the job by helping the body reabsorb the cyst.
- ✿ Through normal eliminative function, the body moves the residue toxin out of the system.

Internal Cleansers

When cysts keep appearing just below the skin, it's time to give the bloodstream a good cleansing. The overall purpose of these regimens is that by cleansing the bloodstream, your child's body will reabsorb the cysts and eliminate them from the body.

- ✿ As you are cleansing your child internally, always be sure that his bowels are moving easily at least once a day, as they are the exit of choice for toxins of all kinds. Chronic skin problems are usually a reflection of toxins that are exiting through the skin, which is precisely what you're trying to avoid. Give him plenty of water to drink, lots of fruits and vegetables to eat, and make sure he gets plenty of exercise. If herbal assistance in elimination is required, see the section on Constipation in Chapter 8.
- ✿ Make red clover, a gentle blood-cleansing herb, a choice treat. You can serve up red clover in a punch made with the tea and your child's favorite juice, or freeze honey-sweetened red clover tea into ice pops. A serving of red clover, in whatever form you and your child choose, may be had three times a day.
- ✿ Echinacea is an excellent blood cleanser and may be given (in addition to the above suggestions) 3 times a day in a little juice. See dosing guidelines in Chapter 3 for amounts appropriate to your child's weight.
- ✿ Most often, it is poor food choices that are polluting your child's bloodstream. Try to engage your child in improving his food options by explaining how the toxic residue of inappropriate foods is hanging out in his bloodstream, causing problems

in his skin. He may look at the next bag of chips with a more
disdainful eye.

BOILS/INFECTED SKIN/PUSTULES

In addition to the above recommendations for internal cleansing,
boils and cysts can be drawn to a head with poultices that draw
infection from the skin.

Drawing Poultices

In a blender, macerate with water, fresh or dried drawing herbs:
comfrey root or leaf, marshmallow root, burdock root, and/or plantain leaf*; with fresh or dried antimicrobial herbs: echinacea root,
or leaves and flowers, and a fresh clove of garlic; or add a few drops
essential oil of thyme to the finished poultice.

- Use only enough water to make the herbs into a mash; you
  don't want the consistency to be runny.
- Start blending the herbs while dry, adding water to moisten
  until a thick, wet mass of herbs is the result. This will break
  down the capillary walls, releasing more of the herbs' healing
  benefits.
- Place the herbal mash on gauze or cheesecloth. Make a little
  packet of it and apply to the affected area.
- Affixing the herbal packet to the skin with roller gauze and surgical tape will hold it in place comfortably.
- Replace the poultice with fresh material 2–3 times a day until
  the area is healed, allowing it to be exposed to the air or sun-
  light for an hour or two between poultice applications.

------

*Almost everyone who has grass growing on the lawn has some plantain grow-
ing, too; just be certain that you correctly identify this plant with an identification guide, and—most vital of all—that the plantain has not been chemically
treated in any way.

✿ You can make enough herbal mash for a whole day at one time. Simply add a little water to rehydrate, if necessary.

Instant Drawing Poultice

A quick-and-easy drawing poultice can be made by combining powdered echinacea root that is moistened into a paste with oil of garlic.

✿ Apply to the affected area, cover with gauze, holding it in place as described above.
✿ Refresh twice a day.

Until you get to the health food store to purchase ingredients for your drawing poultice, a pack of steamed, thinly sliced onions will get the drawing action started.

✿ Steam the onions.
✿ Enclose them in a packet of gauze or cheesecloth.
✿ Affix to the skin as described above.

PSORIASIS

This is yet another skin ailment that reflects the need for internal cleansing and dietary changes.

✿ First, test your child's foods using the method described in Appendix C, eliminating all foods that test poorly.
✿ Herbal ointments containing calendula, comfrey, chickweed, or burdock offer topical relief for psoriasis and may be applied as often as needed.
✿ For internal therapy, look for formulas containing the roots of yellow dock, burdock, sarsaparilla, and dandelion, all of which cleanse the bloodstream. See Chapter 3 for dosing guidelines.
✿ The addition of essential fatty acids (EFAs—Omega 3's and

6's—available in flaxseed oil, borage oil, evening primrose oil, fish oils, and black currant oil) can be important for their anti-inflammatory action. Consult with your local health food store for a formula appropriate for your child.

❂ Finally, as with all skin ailments, make sure your child is having daily bowel movements. See suggestions under "Cysts," above.

SKIN ULCERS

Whenever your child's skin is looking angry and inflamed, a poultice made of slippery elm bark will help to calm it.

❂ Mix the powdered slippery elm with enough warm water to make a paste.

❂ This can be applied by itself, or if you need to add some antimicrobial properties to the poultice, add powdered echinacea or calendula to the slippery elm.

INFLAMED SKIN AND POISON PLANT RASHES

Sometimes, we don't know exactly what has caused the skin to flare up; and while it would be helpful to know (so as to avoid repeated contact), you certainly don't have to know the exact source to use this wonderful, healing poultice.

Soothe-All Poultice

I wouldn't dream of taking my kids on a country outing—or even spending an afternoon in the woods—without the powerfully healing ingredients in this soothing, anti-inflammatory, antimicrobial herbal paste.

❂ Mix equal parts powdered slippery elm bark and goldenseal (one teaspoon to one tablespoon of each should suffice).

- Moisten with water to make a paste and apply to the affected area. More may be applied each day.
- Do not remove the old paste, as the body will reject it when it is ready to do so. Instead, add fresh paste over the old.
- Cover with a bandage both to protect the affected area and to prevent the paste from staining the clothing.

IMPETIGO

Impetigo is a highly contagious bacterial (staph) infection that may appear on its own, or as a secondary infection to another skin affliction. The following remedies work very well:

For external therapy:

- Compress affected areas with combined infusions of antimicrobial herbs such as echinacea, goldenseal, thyme, and myrrh. See Appendix A for guidelines for preparing infusions and compresses.
- Antimicrobial compresses may also be made from the essential oils of tea tree, thyme, and/or eucalyptus.
- Be sure to dry the area thoroughly after compressing.
- Compress area 3–4 times a day for 20 minutes each time.
- You can prepare a soothing, itch-relieving ointment by blending several drops of myrrh liquid extract with a small amount of calendula ointment.

For internal therapy:

- Give your child blood-cleansing herb teas such as red clover or burdock root, 3 times a day.
- Keep the immune system stimulated with doses of echinacea three times a day. See section on Echinacea in Chapter 12 for guidelines.
- Give antimicrobial garlic (fresh cloves, tablets, perles, or oil) 3 times a day.

Anxiety-Reducing Herbs

Perhaps you're wondering why I would be talking about herbs to reduce anxiety in a chapter on skin ailments. I do so because we all react to disturbances in our bodies in different ways. I find I deal with stomach problems with equanimity, while the itch of a single mosquito bite drives me to distraction!

Similarly, some children are not upset by skin ailments, while others become totally frazzled. If your child's skin problem is indeed anxiety-provoking, consider giving nervine herbs (see Chapter 11) and/or Bach Flower Essences (see Appendix I) to help deal with the situation. Your child will invariably heal more quickly if the emotional quotient is not present to exacerbate the skin issue.

Dandruff

Dandruff, if not caused by a hair product, is often the way the skin manifests internal toxins. It may also be a signal to clean up your child's diet. Sage and tea tree can be used as a rinse and shampoo.

- ❧ Steep 2 teaspoons sage leaf in a cup of boiled water until cool.
- ❧ A larger quantity can be stored in the refrigerator for 3 days.
- ❧ Pour through the hair after shampooing; do not rinse out.
- ❧ A shampoo containing tea tree oil may also be helpful. (Commercial shampoos are increasingly using this herb, though the ones you purchase at a health food store are usually better.)
- ❧ A few drops tea tree oil may be added to water and poured through hair; do not rinse out.

FUNGAL INFECTIONS

Fungal infections common to children include athlete's foot, ringworm (a circular rash that can be but is not limited to transmission by cats), nail infections, and ear fungus.

Pau D'Arco

Pau d'arco is a South American herb used for stimulating the body's immune system and as an antimicrobial. Give a dose three times a day (liquid extract, capsule, or tea) to internally support the body in overcoming the fungal infection. (See Chapter 3 for dosing guidelines.)

Tea Tree Oil

Tea tree, native to Australia and easily found in health food stores, contains potent antiseptic and antifungal properties.

- Dilute a few drops tea tree oil in ½–1 teaspoon of a carrier oil such as almond or sunflower, and apply topically 3 or 4 times a day.
- Tea tree oil may be used undiluted but may be too strong for your child's sensitive skin. You may wish to experiment to see what the strongest dilution may be that is well tolerated by decreasing the amount of carrier oil.

Andrea's AntiFungal Oil

This pleasant-smelling, soothing oil can be made ahead and stored in your herbal medicine chest, ready for use at the first sighting of a fungal rash. Apply in the morning and at bedtime.

10 drops tea tree oil
5 drops lavender oil
12 oz almond or sunflower oil

Athlete's Foot Remedy

- ❀ To remedy a mild form of this condition, massage the essential oil of lavender into new occurrences of athlete's foot. (Lavender is one of the few essential oils that may be applied directly to the skin without dilution.)
- ❀ Make sure your child is wearing 100% cotton socks and expose the feet to the air as much as possible.
- ❀ Instruct your child to dry well between the toes after bathing.
- ❀ Natural antifungal foot powders may be found in the health food store.
- ❀ Use the tea tree oil remedy, mentioned above, for more tenacious cases of athlete's foot.

WARM HANDS AND FEET

This is a wonderful way to send your little ones out to play in the snow without worrying that their hands and feet will get cold.

Ginger Hand-and-Foot Warmer

Sprinkle 1–2 teaspoons powdered ginger into your children's mittens and socks. The ginger will bring herbal heat to the extremities and keep them toasty warm!

As long as we're talking about warming the extremities with herbs . . . the heat of cayenne can be used to keep the feet warm.

Cayenne Foot Warmer

If your child is a skier, long days out on the slopes can mean frigid toes. You can put ginger powder in their mittens or gloves and cayenne powder in the socks.

- ❀ For the feet, use cayenne (which has even more herbal heat) by putting 1 tablespoon of the powdered herb in a pair of socks that are put over your child's socks. (This is so that she doesn't touch the cayenne with her fingers, which, if rubbed in the eyes, can cause irritation.)

✿ When your child is ready to undress after the outdoor activity, remove both pairs of socks together and wash.

The Gastrointestinal System

I received the following in an e-mail from RealAge.com (you can subscribe for free to receive helpful health tips), and thought it worth sharing with you. It is, you might say, food for thought.

Want to improve your kids' eating habits? Turn your dinner hour into family hour. Though it might be a challenge to get the whole gang to sit down together, a new study shows that it may be worth the extra effort. Researchers at Harvard Medical School studied the eating habits of 16,000 children and found that the kids who ate dinner with their families consumed more fruits and veggies, fewer fried foods, saturated fats, and trans fats, and more fiber than the youngsters who rarely ate with their folks.

I have yet to meet the otherwise healthy child who has not, at one time or another, suffered from tummyaches, motion sickness, or an occasional bout of the runs.

The remedies I share here are among the easiest and least intimidating to use. And because they're more pleasant than most medicine, your kids will thank you, too.

TUMMYACHES

A simple tummyache can result from many sources: having eaten too quickly, anxiety, or even a need for attention. In all such matters, I have found a cup of the digestive teas, chamomile or peppermint, sweetened with a little honey, to be the comforting answer.

GAS, BLOATING, AND DIGESTIVE UPSET

Food Issues

If this is a recurrent situation with your child, you need to determine which family of foods is the culprit. Wheat (found in pasta, bread, crackers, cookies, pretzels, and cereals) and dairy can cause bloating in many children. Keep a food diary of what your child eats, and you will soon be able to pinpoint the offending foods.

Another approach to identifying offending foods is described in Appendix C.

Yet another approach would be food combining. Based on the concept that proteins take longer for the body to digest than carbohydrates, it is recommended that they be eaten separately. This would mean, for example, that nut butters (proteins) would not be eaten on bread (carbohydrates) because their rate of digestion would differ. Similarly, fruits, which are digested quickly, would be eaten by themselves. If fruit is eaten directly before, during, or after a protein meal, its digestion would be delayed allowing for fermentation in the body, leading to gas and bloating. For a thorough explanation of food combining see John and Marilyn Diamond's book, *Fit for Life*.

Herbal Support

Until you figure out which foods to eliminate from your child's diet, try using acidophilus (the active culture in yogurt) 3 times a day, to promote healthier intestinal flora, as well as one of the following teas, as needed, for their antispasmodic, antiflatulent properties:

Peppermint
Ginger
Sage
Fennel seed
Dill seed
See Appendix A for how to prepare medicinal herb teas and
    Chapter 3 for dosing guidelines.

Honegar

Gas and bloating are often due to an acid/alkaline imbalance resulting from improperly digested foods, food sensitivities, or stress. The wonderful tonic that follows helps restore equilibrium to your child's digestive system.

Mix 1 tablespoon apple cider vinegar and 1 teaspoon honey (both are best purchased in the health food store for the most natural versions) into ½ cup water. Serve in ¼–½ cup doses at room temperature, or heated as a tea. You can repeat this dosage several times a day if necessary.

DIARRHEA

Diarrhea may be a manifestation of a food intolerance, a passing virus or, if an ongoing problem, may signal a deeper infection, or the presence of parasites. In addition to taking action appropriate to its cause, the following suggestions may provide immediate relief.

Herbal Teas, Tablets, and Oil

This is a good time for a discussion of the intriguing sage leaf. Sage is a diaphoretic herb. This means that when it is taken hot, it increases the flow of fluids; and, when taken cold, it decreases them.

It is this diaphoretic property and its astringency that make sage an excellent remedy for diarrhea when taken as a cold tea.

- ❀ Make a quart of sage tea by steeping 4 to 6 teaspoons sage leaf in a quart of boiled water until cool; strain.
- ❀ Encourage your child to take frequent sips throughout the day, or until the bowels are normalized.

When else would you want to shut down fluids? Just ask a menopausal woman with hot flashes! Cold sage tea brings welcome relief. When you want to sweat out a cold or flu, hot sage tea is a good way to help flush out toxins through perspiration.

- ❀ Another good tea for stopping diarrhea is raspberry leaf. High in tannins, its astringency helps curtail diarrhea and can be sipped warm.
- ❀ If your child has pain and discomfort along with the diarrhea, the addition of peppermint leaf to the raspberry leaf tea may help due to its antispasmodic action on the smooth muscle of the digestive tract.
- ❀ Slippery elm bark is a soothing, anti-inflammatory herb. In addition to astringent teas, you may have your child suck on tablets made of slippery elm (available in health food stores). For the child who is too young to suck on a tablet, see the slippery elm recommendations in the section on diarrhea in Chapter 9.
- ❀ A soothing oil which you can gently massage into the baby's or child's stomach area can be made from a few drops essential oil of chamomile diluted in 1 teaspoon vegetable or nut oil. This can be repeated 3–4 times a day, if needed. In this form, chamomile's digestive benefits are absorbed through the skin.

Food Recommendations

Until the child's bowels have calmed down, I recommend brown rice, plain yogurt, blueberries, and banana—any combination that provides the most pleasant texture and taste. You can flavor these foods with a bit of honey and/or cinnamon.

In addition, vegetable broth and lots of water will help prevent dehydration and will restore the electrolyte balance in your child's body.

Acidophilus, which is the concentrated form of the active culture in yogurt, can be given 3 or 4 times a day to balance the intestinal flora, which in some cases helps eliminate the diarrhea at its source.

For infant diarrhea, see Chapter 9, "Baby's Comfort."

CONSTIPATION

I have learned that constipation is defined differently by almost as many different people as I ask. For some, this means not moving the bowels at least once a day; for others, every three days. If this were a medical pop quiz, the former answer would be correct.

Here's one way to think of it. The average human body temperature is, as you know, 98.6 degrees Fahrenheit. At the risk of being too graphic, picture a piece of meat sitting on your kitchen counter overnight in the heat of summer. I'm sure you wouldn't want it in your child's body. The bottom line is that what your child eats today should be easily passed out of the body tomorrow. That translates into having at least one bowel movement a day.

Natural Remedies

If your child is constipated, I recommend the following approaches:

- ✿ Prune juice, diluted with an equal part water, with the juice of one-half lemon works well to get the system moving.
- ✿ High-fiber cereal eaten before bedtime also works well.
- ✿ Flaxseed is a good intestinal lubricant and helpful in chronic constipation. Consider adding ½–1 teaspoon flaxseed oil to your child's food once or twice a day, on an ongoing basis (it mixes well in mashed potatoes, vegetables, salads, on toast).

However, as this oil can turn rancid quickly, it is important that you buy it fresh from your local health food store's refrigerated section. Always smell it before serving to be sure it still has a fresh, nutty taste.

Interestingly, flaxseed has been cultivated since at least 5000 BC: Hippocrates recommended its use to his fellow Greeks, and Charlemagne mandated its use to the 18th-century French. Mahatma Gandhi said, "Wherever flax seeds become a regular food item among the people, there will be better health."

- Acidophilus restores the balance of intestinal flora; thus, just as it helps diarrhea, so, too, does acidophilus help the child who tends toward constipation.
- Plain yogurt is a good food for the constipated child, and works especially well when you add pureed prunes, figs, or applesauce. An easy source of pureed food is commercial baby food, even if your child is too old to eat baby food!
- Herbal formulations are readily available in health food stores. Look for those that include: cascara sagrada, fennel, turkey rhubarb, and ginger. Give at bedtime as they take several hours to gently stimulate peristaltic action in the colon.
- Avoid preparations that include the herb senna—it is found in many laxative teas, but it is too harsh for children.
- I especially recommend Dr. Christopher's Fen (for fennel) LB (for lower bowel) formula; it can be found in capsule, liquid, or tablet form. I do not recommend relying on a lower-bowel formula daily, but rest assured that this formula is not at all addictive when used as an occasional (once or twice a week if absolutely necessary) adjunct to a good diet and lots of water. The flip side of this is that rather than live a "constipated life," in spite of a good diet and lots of water, your child would do better to take Fen LB more, rather than less, frequently.
- Emotional stress and travel can throw off anyone's normal bowel habits, and Fen LB helps wonderfully to restore balance.
- Whenever you give any herbal bowel formula, be sure to give

your child lots of water to drink along with the dose to help activate it.

  ❀ Slippery elm bark can provide gentle help for constipation. Give your child a capsule 2 or 3 times a day. Alternately, you can make a tea from the bark (see the section on herbal decoctions in Appendix A); give your child ½ cup doses. You can also prepare a cereal from slippery elm (see section on diarrhea in Chapter 9).

  ❀ Sometimes, water is the only "remedy" required to relieve chronic constipation. Other liquids are not suitable replacements! My children were brought up with water as the first beverage to go to for thirst, as have children in France, Italy, and much of the rest of the world. Of course, they liked soda and juice, but these were usually had as a special treat, an "entertainment for their taste buds."

  ❀ The stimulating properties of ginger are also good for the bowels. I keep ginger syrup on hand as a flavoring for seltzer water, so that I can make a quick and delicious natural ginger ale for guests. (Of course, you realize by now that I don't keep soda in my house.) Little do my friends know they are actually getting a good bowel tonic as well!

Dairy and Constipation

Intolerance to dairy products commonly produces diarrhea. Interestingly, the result can, instead, be constipation. Researchers discovered that dairy can produce anal fissures in some children. The pain the fissures caused upon elimination produced a fear of bowel movements leading to constipation. Substitution with soy milk produced a healing of the fissures and, consequently, no more constipation.

STOMACH CRAMPS

The antispasmodic properties of a ginger compress offer a gentle, soothing treatment for stomach cramps. See Gentle Ginger Compress in Chapter 10.

IRRITABLE BOWEL SYNDROME/COLITIS

These intestinal syndromes can manifest as a variety of gastrointestinal symptoms. Adding enteric-coated peppermint oil capsules to your child's preventative health regime may be helpful. If the diet has been changed, and more than the above-mentioned remedies is needed, consider creating a formula of antispasmodic, soothing, and calming herbs.

Antispasmodics: chamomile, peppermint, wild yam root, ginger root

Soothing: slippery elm bark, marshmallow root, comfrey (See Appendix H for a special note on comfrey.)

Calming: chamomile, valerian.

- ❧ By purchasing these herbs in liquid-extract form, you can prepare a stock extract of a combination appropriate to your child's needs.
- ❧ Don't be afraid to experiment with the mixture. Any and all of the above herbs can be combined.
- ❧ Decide, according to herbs' respective properties, which your child needs most, including more of those herbs in the mixture you prepare. See Chapter 3 for dosing guidelines on how many drops of the liquid extract should be given to your child.
- ❧ Give this formula 3 or 4 times a day, diluted in a small amount of water or juice.

NAUSEA/MOTION SICKNESS

Whether from motion sickness or the stomach flu, there are several excellent natural therapies to address the uncomfortable symptoms of nausea.

Peppermint Oil

Oil of peppermint is an effective remedy for nausea. If your oil of peppermint is of high quality, it would be wise to have your child close her eyes as she sips; otherwise, its potency may irritate them.

- ⚘ Simply inhaling this essential oil straight from its bottle helps, as does sipping peppermint tea.
- ⚘ My favorite way to make an instant antinausea tea is to add one drop oil of peppermint (not two drops!) to one cup warm water. Inhaling the tea (for its antinausea, aromatherapeutic properties) as well as sipping it will help settle your child's stomach, and relieve queasiness and nausea.

Motion Sickness Tea

Ginger root, when compared in controlled tests to leading pharmaceutical antinausea preparations, has been found to be equally as effective, without the side effects of some pharmaceuticals.

- ⚘ The ginger root can be prepared as a tea from the fresh root (see Appendix A for preparation of a decoction) or can be taken in capsules (1–2 capsule doses).
- ⚘ Give the ginger root to your child 20 minutes prior to travel, 20 minutes after travel is in progress, and another 20 minutes later if nausea is still present.

The Throw-Up Button!

In my home, this is what we call the acupressure point that relieves nausea.

I once used this point on the passenger sitting next to me during a bumpy plane ride. It spared us both the unpleasant consequences of her motion sickness. I've even used it in the bathroom of a restaurant on a pregnant woman who was suffering from morning sickness. Teaching this point to your children may help them to get to the bathroom when they feel the urge to throw up.

- ✿ Place the index and middle fingers of your right hand on top of the "knob" of the child's right clavicle bone in the neck area.
- ✿ Slide your fingers into the hollow along the inside of the bone and hold firmly for several minutes. It may be sensitive at first, but this will pass. (See figure #4.)

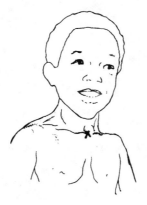

HICCOUGHS

My method of chasing away hiccoughs has impressed even the most skeptical parent.

- ✿ Using both index fingers, firmly hold the child's parotid glands, which are located in the hollow behind the ear lobes. (See figure #5.)
- ✿ Keep a firm pressure on these points while he drinks as much water as he can without stopping. By the time he finishes drinking, his hiccoughs will have disappeared.

❀ A nursing or bottle-fed infant's hiccoughs can be relieved in
the same way.

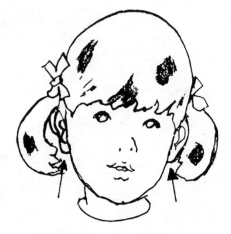

PARASITES AND WORMS

If your child is diagnosed with parasites or worms, become a detective to determine where the infestation is coming from so you
can stop this condition from returning once you have treated it.
Sometimes this is difficult, as the parasites/worms can come from
food eaten in a restaurant. The important thing is this: Don't panic!
Try, for peace of mind for both of you, to disassociate your image of
creepy crawlies with your child's condition. Our bodies are bom-
barded with microscopic organisms every day of our lives; worms
and parasites are just another form of these.

If you are dealing with pinworms or threadworms, an aggressive
washing of bed linens is required; additionally, you should isolate
your child's towels from those used by the rest of the family. For these
parasites, in addition to the garlic remedy discussed below, I have
found a homeopathic remedy of threadworm (made by Hanna's
Herb Shop) to be most helpful. (See Appendix G for resources.)

Also, do keep in mind that sugar feeds parasites. While it's always
a good idea, this is the perfect time to reduce your child's sugar

intake. Remember, too, that juice (which is often thought to be so "healthy") is just another form of sugar.

The herb world contains many antiparasitical plants, but I have found that the common kitchen herb, garlic, is the very best of all.

The Glorious Garlic Go-Fer

This remedy earns its name because garlic "goes fer" parasites in a big way!

- ✿ Once a day, for three days, add 1 tablespoon chopped fresh garlic to your child's food.
- ✿ It is delicious when added to mashed potatoes, spread on buttered toast (for an impromptu garlic bread), and on pasta (especially with olive oil).
- ✿ One week after the third garlic treatment, repeat the 3-day treatment.
- ✿ Wait one week and repeat once again.
- ✿ The weeks in between allow any residual parasites to hatch, after which you can once again zap them with the garlic.
- ✿ During this treatment period, be sure to give your child plenty of water, plus fibrous foods to make sure the bowels are moving well daily.

HEARTBURN

Heartburn, or acid reflux, seems to be a problem of almost epidemic proportions these days—one that some people think requires the daily use of medication to counteract it. I've even learned that infants are being put on medication for excessive spitting up. When heartburn occurs in teenagers and adults, it is often attributed to stress—but in infants? Yes, an infant's digestive processes could reflect the tension in a baby's environment, though it is far more likely that eating too fast or not burping a baby sufficiently can contribute to this problem. But the question remains: Is medication the solution, or is it simply masking this problem's underlying cause?

Based upon my observations, it seems that unless there is a distinct physiological stimulus for acid reflux—such as a hiatal hernia—the cause usually lies in food intake and unrecognized dehydration, especially in infants.

Dehydration

For the nursing infant, acid reflux may relate to the mother's diet as well as dehydration. Infants are not usually given frequent sips of water; instead, they are either nursed or given bottles of formula or juice. For older children, the drinks of choice are most often soda, juice, and sometimes, even coffee! Water is usually considered nothing more than the substance that washes down the morning vitamin or what one drinks when no sugared beverage is around. In Europe, conversely, water remains for most people the beverage of choice (though the tens of millions of dollars spent annually on advertising by huge cola companies is, I fear, changing this pattern even in France, the very source of premium bottled water).

Food Intake

I have often found that heartburn in children is the result of overindulgence or of poor food choices. Eating too fast, or while under stress, also compromises digestion and can cause acid reflux. Often, just sipping a glass of room-temperature water is enough to soothe the unpleasant sensation. If the heartburn is experienced while in bed, elevate your child's head and upper body with extra pillows.

Today, Americans eat more carbohydrates (pasta, breads, baked goods, snack foods) than ever before. HIgh-carbohydrate foods turn to sugar in the body, thus upsetting our natural acid/alkaline balance. Further, many of them are laden with chemicals. Reducing children's intake of these white-floured foods does much to diminish acid reflux when this has been problematic.

Natural Solutions

The solution? My clients of all ages have been able to resolve the acid reflux/heartburn issue without medication by incorporating the following, very simple recommendations:

1. Drink lots of water.
   - Make nature's own beverage the only drink available with and between meals.
   - It is difficult for the body to take in large amounts of chilled water, so give your child room-temperature water. Besides, if the water is standing out on the kitchen counter, you and your child are more likely to remember to drink it.
   - Encourage your child to drink before and after physical activity. Put a bottle of water in your child's school backpack so that it is always available. Soon you will find that the more a child drinks, the thirstier he gets!
   - Make the drinking of water a habit in your home. We did in mine, and to this day it is what my sons and I choose to drink. (Sure, I let them have the occasional soda as a treat—when outside our home—but it was not an item that was included in our weekly shopping.)
2. Give your child's body an opportunity to return to its proper acid/alkaline balance by:
   - Reducing carbohydrate intake (sugary snacks, pastry, cookies, fruit juice, crackers, bread, pasta, puddings). They don't have to be totally eliminated but in reducing the greater offenders like candy and cookies, small amounts of bread and pasta would be better tolerated.
   - Replacing them with protein foods (fish, chicken, meat, soy products, vegetables, eggs, nuts).
   - When you make these dietary changes, you'll soon realize how unbalanced your child's present food intake really is.
   - You can reintroduce carbohydrates, keeping them reasonably balanced with proteins, when the acid reflux is no longer an issue.

3. Herbs can also provide temporary relief for acid reflux.
    • Aloe juice, available in virtually every health food store, is a
      gentle restorer of the body's pH. Mix ¼ to ½ teaspoon in ¼ to
      ½ cup water and give to your child 3 times a day.
    • Slippery elm bark, powdered and encapsulated or mixed
      with water, can be given as a cereal; you may flavor it with
      cinnamon. Give your child one capsule or the cereal 3
      times a day unless she suffers from loose bowel movements,
      in which case you should reduce the dose to once or twice a
      day. Soothing relief nearly always ensues.
    • Spearmint tea is a fine remedy for the occasional bout of
      heartburn, but if it's an ongoing problem it needs to be
      addressed with an ongoing plan to prevent it from occurring
      in the first place.

9

Baby's Comfort

Is anything more important to a parent than making sure our newborn is as safe, content, and as comfortable as can be? No matter how many times our doctor tells us baby is crying to get food, attention, or to be changed, we always think our baby is telling us more. If we only knew what baby wanted, we would do anything to soothe their spirits . . . but, alas, all we hear are cries. (And of course, in just a few years, our child will be vocalizing just a bit too much!)

I love talking about these wonderful, super-safe herbal remedies for infants because from cradle cap to diaper rash, the everyday discomforts of infancy respond beautifully to these effective yet gentle natural applications.

DIAPER RASH

When my boys were babies, my friends and family thought my choice of baby supplies rather odd. Instead of the cute, sweet-smelling products marketed to parents, I preferred to use substances that were free of harsh additives, as well as nourishing and healing to my babies' skin.

Tender Skin-Cleansing Herbs for Baby

Do you have fond, aromatic memories of a relative who smelled of delicate rose water wherever she went? Your baby can have a signature scent, too. You can create an aromatic, antimicrobial cleansing water that is perfect for washing the tender diaper area—and your baby will smell good, too.

- Add several drops essential oil of lavender, rosemary, calendula, or rose to a pint of distilled water, and—voila! You now have a skin-loving, antimicrobial wash that's totally chemical-free.
- You can cut a supply of squares from a cotton diaper to use as cloths for cleansing baby's bottom (which can then be washed and reused); or, if you prefer, purchase disposable cotton pads.

Herbs for Soothing Diaper Rash

Why use additive-laden treatments when you can purchase totally natural ones, prepared in a base of olive oil and beeswax, that are wonderfully soothing and healing for even the tenderest skin? Check out your health food store or see Appendices G and H for resources and product ingredients.

Look for anti-inflammatory, astringent, and antimicrobial ingredients such as chamomile, chickweed, comfrey, marshmallow root, mullein leaf, and black walnut.

Powder Protection

Powdered slippery elm bark makes an excellent powder for the tender diaper area. It is best to avoid commercial products containing talc, mineral oil, or fragrances. If you suspect an overgrowth of yeast in your child's system (see pages 208–210), giving acidophilus will help restore balance to the intestinal tract. For further discussion of herbs for yeast tissues, see the section on fungus.

One other tip: If you like the texture of baby powder but don't want your baby to experience the potentially harmful effects of talc, use cornstarch right from the box on the diaper area.

An Ounce of Prevention

☘ The lovely, yellow flowers of St. John's Wort and mullein can be infused in olive oil to nourish the skin while providing antimicrobial and anti-inflammatory protection for baby. These oils can be purchased in the health food store and combined, at home, in one bottle.

☘ To make your own skin-nurturing, antimicrobial herbal oil, add several drops essential oil of lavender or chamomile to an 8 ounce bottle of cold-pressed almond, apricot kernel, or grapeseed oil.

Recurrent or intense rashes in the diaper area need to be investigated for probable cause.

Always buy natural, chemical-free cloth diapers. Be certain that you wash diapers in mild soap that is chemical- and fragrance-free. Know that rubber pants worn over cloth diapers will worsen rashes by keeping the area moist.

If you use disposables, it is possible that your baby's rash may be the result of an allergy to the composition of synthetic disposable material. If you have your heart set on using disposables, you can try changing the diapers more frequently—and leave them off entirely when appropriate.

Your child's diet may need to be tested for offending foods. If you are a nursing mother, you should examine your own diet. Consider commonly allergenic foods like dairy, wheat, corn, peanuts, chocolate, eggs, and refined sugar.

THRUSH, CANDIDA, AND YEAST

These conditions all derive from the same microorganism: fungus. Thrush, which is white with underlying red patches found in a baby's mouth, indicates a fungal infection from mouth to anus. See page 209 for further discussion.

You can clear up thrush by giving baby oral doses of antifungal herbs while the infection is active and up to 10 days after it clears. In addition to ridding the body of fungus, this treatment will help strengthen baby's immune system. See Chapter 3 for dosing guidelines.

Garlic oil (3 or 4 times a day)
Echinacea extract (4 times a day)
Black walnut extract (twice a day)
Acidophilus (4 times a day) (See page 210.)

CRADLE CAP

A form of seborrheic dermatitis, cradle cap is a skin inflammation reflecting internal disharmony.

Natural Approaches (Internal)

- Adding acidophilus, the active culture in yogurt, to baby's diet will help restore healthful intestinal flora. (See page 210.)
- It is also important to check both mother's and baby's diet for food allergies, which can contribute to the internal toxicity.
- Blood-cleansing herbs such as burdock root, dandelion root, red clover flower, and nettle leaf—in any combination—given to a nursing mother or to the newborn will help clear impurities from the bloodstream, thus helping clear cradle cap. See Chapter 3 for dosing guidelines.

Natural Approaches (Topical)

- At bedtime, saturate baby's scalp with nourishing and moisturizing castor oil or olive oil mixed with a few drops of antimicrobial oil of rosemary.

- In the morning, massage baby's scalp with the residue oil, comb through, and remove the dry matter.
- During the day, apply chamomile cream or St. John's Wort oil. Both are skin-healing, anti-inflammatory herbs that work wonders on cradle cap.

Comfrey Root Scalp Rinse

- After a nightly shampooing, rinse baby's head with comfrey root tea.
- Prepare a decoction (see Appendix A for preparation); cool until just warm.
- Pour the tea through baby's head; do not wash out; gently pat to remove excess moisture.
- Allow the mucilaginous comfrey to air-dry in baby's scalp. Comfrey is noted for its ability to encourage the growth of healthy skin.

GENERAL SKIN CARE

Cleansing Baths

The common dilemma: you seek the antimicrobial benefits of soaps but without chemical ingredients.

The solution: herbal baths, which leave a lovely, natural aroma on the skin while providing antimicrobial cleansing action.

- For a wonderful herbal bath, add a quart of an herbal infusion (see Appendix A for preparation guidelines) of chamomile, lavender, rosemary, or calendula to baby's bath water.
- Alternatively, you can add 2 to 3 drops of one of these herbs' essential oils directly to the water.
- If you desire more cleansing power, fill a muslin bag with oatmeal, moisten it with the herb-filled bathwater, and wash hard-to-clean parts of baby's body that need extra cleansing action.

Moisturizing Herbs

Why use a moisturizer laden with overbearing fragrances, chemicals, and preservatives when nature has such a wonderful moisturizer: almond oil? If you desire a natural fragrance, add a few drops essential oil of lavender to 8 ounces almond oil. The result is a lovely aroma that soothes baby as well as you!

Look in your local health food store for creams that contain moisturizing herbs such as chickweed, calendula, comfrey, and chamomile.

COLIC

Every new parent feels helpless when baby cries, so we have to do a bit of investigative work to find out what the problem is and how we can make our newborn more comfortable. If his legs are drawn up to the stomach and baby seems in pain, the problem could very well be gas pains.

Because colic is related to digestion, examine baby's food intake to try to determine the source of the gas. Perhaps baby's formula needs to be changed. Quite often, newborns have an intolerance to cow's milk. However, before you make baby go through the allergy-testing process, I recommend using the surrogate muscle-testing method presented in Appendix C.

In many cases, the nursing mother is ingesting gas-producing foods. If mother limits her intake of these foods, baby's colic may well disappear.

Check to see if baby is taking in too much air while nursing. In the same vein, be sure to give baby enough time to burp during and after feeding. Elevating baby's head while feeding may relieve digestive discomfort.

Indigestion can be the result of tension in the environment. The information I provide on Bach Flower Essences in Appendix I can help your baby's nervous system cope with the turbulent energy in the air. Another effective approach is to make a concerted effort to create a time of quiet and calm for you and your baby while he feeds. Soft music, be it classical, folk, or New Age, can be very helpful to both of you. By the same token, if someone else is feeding your baby, suggest ways the caregiver can make it a quiet time for the both of them.

Herbal Digestive Aids: Teas and Baths

To relax baby's tummy and help improve digestion, give the follow-ing carminative (digestive) herbs a try to see which works best. They help reduce spasms and inflammation of the digestive tract as well as intestinal gas.

- Before feeding, give your baby a teaspoon of chamomile, fennel seed, or lemon balm tea diluted in one teaspoon distilled water.
- A few sips of diluted peppermint tea helps reduce flatulence.
- Balancing intestinal flora helps maintain a healthier digestive tract. Give baby (and nursing mother) acidophilus twice a day. There are powdered acidophilus products designed specifi-cally for infants available in the health food store.
- A quieting bath can help baby relax muscles and release gas. Add a couple of drops of the essential oils of chamomile and lavender to baby's bath water, or fill a muslin bag with dried lavender and chamomile flowers, and let soak in bath water. The muslin bag can be used to gently sponge baby's body. (Muslin bath bags can be ordered from Frontier—see Appendix G for resource.)

Tummy Intestinal Massage and Compress

Massaging baby's stomach ever so gently helps tummy problems of all kinds.

- Make a wonderful, calming massage oil by blending one drop essential oil of chamomile or lavender in a teaspoon of almond oil.
- In your massage, follow the path of intestinal action—up the baby's right side, across the middle section of the stomach, and down the left side. (See figure #6.)

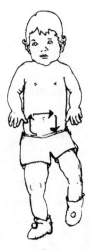

❀ To help calm baby and expel gas, pour 2 tablespoons castor oil
   into a cup; then, place the cup in a saucepan of hot water to
   warm it.

❀ Lay baby on his back, on your stomach, or on bed in front of
   you, with the top of his head facing you. (See figure #7.)

❀ Do a gentle clockwise massage as described above, repeating
   the motion for several minutes.

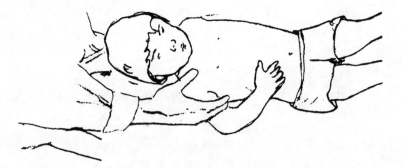

Ginger Compress

Ginger tea is a marvelous stomach restorer in that it relaxes spasms, relieves gas, and stimulates bowel function.

- ❀ Prepare a cup of ginger tea according to directions in Appendix A for preparing a decoction.
- ❀ Cool the tea with an ice cube until it's just warm.
- ❀ Dip a cotton cloth in the tea and compress baby's stomach.
- ❀ Cover with a hot water bottle to keep compress warm.

CONSTIPATION

If your parental intuition tells you that baby's chronic constipation is emotionally based, Bach Flower Essences may be all the infant needs. (See Appendix I). Keep in mind that children are like sponges: if the emotional energy of the family is tense and disturbed, your baby's constipation may be a reflection of this discord.

- ❀ Baby should drink lots of water, nature's own answer to constipation.
- ❀ Pureed figs and/or prunes help maintain regularity.
- ❀ I heartily recommend Dr. Christopher's liquid formula, Fen LB, as a gentle promoter of peristaltic action in the colon. (See Appendix G for information on how to obtain this formula.)

Yeast infections and parasites can also contribute to constipation. If your baby has been diagnosed with either of these microorganisms, see section on herbal remedies for yeast (pages 208–210).

DIARRHEA

Experience with my sons, Brian and Chris, taught me that diarrhea is the easiest imbalance to regulate. At the first sign of diarrhea:

- ❀ I increased their intake of water to guard against dehydration; and
- ❀ fed them mashed, ripened banana to regulate the bowels.

Natural Aids

If your baby's diarrhea is severe and chronic, be on the lookout for food intolerances. These can be in the baby's own system or transmitted through nursing. (See Appendix C for directions on surrogate testing for food sensitivities.)

- ❀ Acidophilus is a wonderful and easy way to balance intestinal flora. A liquid form of acidophilus can be found in health food stores and can be given three to four times a day.
- ❀ Raspberry leaf is an astringent herb that helps stop diarrhea. Its high mineral content is also beneficial to baby's general health. To make this tea, steep one teaspoon of raspberry leaf in a cup of boiled water until cool. Give to the infant by the dropperful, every half an hour until diarrhea stops.
- ❀ Slippery elm bark soothes as it nourishes. You can buy it in powdered form and make a cereal by stirring the herb into warm water until a smooth consistency is reached. Add carob, powdered cinnamon, and/or honey to make this more palatable to a toddler's taste buds.
- ❀ Rosemary is astringent as well as antispasmodic. If your baby seems to be experiencing cramping along with the diarrhea, prepare rosemary tea by simmering a teaspoon of the herb in a cup of water for 15 minutes. In an acute stage, give a dropperful every 15 minutes, then give 2 ounces every one to two hours until symptoms are relieved.
- ❀ Creamed brown rice, mixed with plain yogurt, provides additional nourishment and stool support.
- ❀ Powdered carob (a cocoalike flavoring found in all health food stores) has a rich history of use in controlling diarrhea, and can be added to the slippery elm cereal or the creamed brown rice.

🌼 Countries around the world use foods as medicine. In Sweden, researchers have found that the chemical constituents in blueberries kill bacteria. Swedish physicians treat childhood diarrhea with ⅓-ounce dried blueberries made into a soup.

🌼 If a virus, bacterial infection, or parasite is to blame, try giving garlic oil internally.

VOMITING

For babies, a bit of spitting up after a meal is normal. If, however, your baby is experiencing projectile vomiting, be sure to seek immediate medical care.

Vomiting can sometimes be the result of incompletely digested food; this may be due to food intolerances. Eliminate the offending food and see if the vomiting is curtailed. (See Appendix C for help in determining the offending food.)

Natural Aids

When your baby vomits due to illness:

🌼 Be sure to keep his body well-hydrated by continually offering water and/or diluted herbal teas.

🌼 Infusions of chamomile, dill, fennel, or lemon balm help settle baby's stomach.

🌼 Often, when food cannot be tolerated, slippery elm cereal provides a soothing, healing, and nourishing form of sustenance. Mix the powdered herb with warm water as described above, and feed baby a few teaspoonsful.

OOZING EYES

A little mucus oozing from the eyes, or crusty eyes, can be the result of the body's natural attempt to throw off toxins. If it is not a serious situation requiring medical care, chamomile works quite well to externally cleanse baby's eyes.

- ❧ Prepare an infusion of chamomile (see Appendix A for directions on how to prepare an herbal infusion). Allow to cool; strain.
- ❧ Pour a little of the tea on a cotton pad, and use to gently cleanse baby's outer lids, making sure to use a fresh pad before touching the other eye.
- ❧ If baby's eyes are extremely crusty, wait until she is asleep and compress the eyes with cotton pads or gauze dipped in the cooled chamomile tea.
- ❧ The herbal tea will keep three days in the refrigerator.

PINKEYE/CONJUNCTIVITIS

Please know that pinkeye is extremely contagious. Take precautions not to allow it to spread to you, baby's other caregivers, or other members of your family. Caution others not to touch baby's face and to wash their hands after handling baby or her linens.

Chamomile is an anti-inflammatory, antibacterial herb. Its chemical constituents also promote healing of tissue. These properties make it an excellent choice for healing pink eye.

- ❧ Allow a cup of chamomile tea to completely cool.
- ❧ Strain very well through layers of cloth or a coffee filter so that the tea is completely clear.
- ❧ Using an eyedropper, put 2 drops of the chamomile tea in each eye, 3 times a day.
- ❧ The tea can be refrigerated for up to three days.
- ❧ If at the end of three days the eyes are not completely clear (review Andrea's Rule of Three; see page 3), seek medical help.

FEVERS

Modern medicine's approach to fever is to suppress it. While it is true that extremely high fevers can lead to irreversible damage, be aware that fever is the body's natural way of fighting infection. As such, it is a classic example of how the immune system works.

When baby has a fever, keep him well hydrated with plenty of water. In many cases, a high fever is the body's response to dehydration.

Fever-Reducing Infusions

- ✿ Infusions of chamomile, yarrow, lemon balm, and elderflower help promote perspiration; this, in turn, cools the body, thus reducing baby's fever. (See Appendix A for directions for making herbal infusions.)
- ✿ Give your child a dropperful of any of these herbal infusions every 15 minutes.
- ✿ Increase dose to ¼ cup every 1–2 hours as the fever comes down.
- ✿ When baby's temperature is normal, continue to give him infusions 3 to 4 times a day for three more days to support the recuperation.
- ✿ This is a good time to give echinacea for its immune-stimulating properties and garlic for its ability to fight viral and bacterial infections.

Elderberry Syrup

Another remedy that works wonders is elderberry syrup. Elder flowers are naturally high in vitamin C and other beneficial compounds that help the body throw off toxins; as such, they are good for a variety of symptoms of cold and flu, including runny nose, muscle aches, fever, and sore throat. Scientific study of the extract of the flowers reveals that elder may be effective in protecting the body from the effects of certain strains of flu virus, and can hasten recovery.

Give your child ½ teaspoon, diluted in an ounce of water, several times a day.

Fever-Reducing Baths/Compresses

Warm herbal baths help cool down baby's body.

- ✿ Add 1–2 drops essential oil of chamomile, lavender, or peppermint to the bath water, or use the fresh or dried form of the herbs to make a quart of infusion.
- ✿ If you feel uncomfortable about bathing baby at this time, the same teas or essential oils can be used as compresses on the forehead, back, chest, and feet.

Cell Salts

Ferr. Phos. helps stimulate the body's ability to fight infection. (See Appendix F for additional cell-salt remedies that help bring down fever.)

TEETHING

Some babies go through their teething stages without a murmur, while others suffer (along with you!) as every new tooth comes in. These herbal remedies will help all of you sleep more easily.

Herbal Teething Calmer

- ✿ Compress baby's swollen gums with gauze pads soaked in soothing, cold chamomile tea.
- ✿ You may wish to keep a frozen supply of these tea pads for fast relief.
- ✿ For especially fretful babies, give a dropperful of warm chamomile tea several times throughout the day.

Cell Salts

When teething is accompanied by drooling, the cell salt Nat. Mur. may offer relief. (See Appendix F for more information about cell salts.)

VACCINATION REACTIONS

Whether or not to vaccinate babies and children is the subject of ongoing debate between mainstream medicine and holistically minded parents. If you are considering going against the prevailing medical tide, you must educate yourself well. As a parent, the decision is up to you, but it must be a responsible and confident one.

Whether you choose to immunize your baby or not, I suggest you bring your child to a doctor who employs homeopathy as part of his or her practice. Properly used, homeopathic preparations, another form of holistic therapy, can protect your baby postimmunization.

Preparing for Vaccinations

If you do choose to immunize your children, consider providing the most ideal environment, both internally and externally, for the event. In addition:

- Be sure your child is well nourished and in excellent health at the time of the inoculation.
- Strengthen baby's immune system with echinacea and vitamin C prior to the vaccination appointment.
- If your baby is teething, wait until symptoms have passed.
- Make absolutely certain your child is not exposed to anyone else's illness, pre- and post-vaccination.

If your child responds to immunization with any untoward, severe reactions—including high fever, seizures, twitching, and extreme emotional responses, seek medical attention immediately, both conventional *and* homeopathic.

Calming Pre-Injection Jitters

For the child who is old enough to develop pre-injection anxiety, Bach Flower Rescue Remedy can be quite calming. (See Appendix I for more information.) The remedy may be given at home, prior to the doctor's visit, and at the office—both before and after injection.

The Magic of Castor Oil

When my children received immunizations, I applied castor oil to the site of the injection, and it always prevented localized inflammatory reactions. Mothers have called me with screaming babies on their laps after a vaccination. Following my suggestion, they would immediately apply castor oil to the site of the injection. The babies would calm down, and the redness and inflammation would reduce while we were still on the phone!

If Vaccination Is Followed by Fever

- ☙ The fever that sometimes accompanies vaccination can be reduced with oral doses of white willow bark (known as herbal aspirin, since white willow bark is the plant upon which aspirin is based).
- ☙ Another fever reducer is a sponge bath with essential oils of peppermint or chamomile. See the section on fever for further suggestions for reducing your child's temperature.

An Extra Dose for Peace of Mind

An effective way of removing excess toxins that the vaccination may leave is to give your child the homeopathic remedy Thuja in 6X potency, twice daily for 2 to 3 weeks following the injection(s).

10

Herbal Programs for the Teen Years

Ask any physician, psychologist—and, yes, any parent—and they will tell you that there is more physical and spiritual upheaval during the teen years than at any other time of our lives. Hormones are part of this, of course, but endocrinology tells only half the story. The other half is that the socialization process during adolescence is in many ways a microcosm of our entire lives, and foreshadows who we are to become. This powerful combination of personality and biology is intense and exciting (I just love listening to impassioned teens discussing everything from a meal to a date to a new CD), yet it manifests in a variety of untoward ways, many of which can be assuaged with the use of herbs.

When he was around 13 years old, Andy was going through a particularly stressful time that resulted in unpredictable emotional outbursts. He wasn't a happy camper, and was not interested in eating healthfully any more. Sugar and junk food were his foods of choice. His pH was out of whack due to the toxic effects of stress hormones and the toxins from the foods he was ingesting.

I recommended the Honegar formula, described below, in hopes of restoring his chemical balance. The results: even as Andy continued to deal with the emotional turmoil of the household, the Honegar seemed to calm his rage as well as his craving for junk food. Honegar: a simple combination of apple cider vinegar and honey—a safe, chemical-free way to keep the peace! Not as surprising a solution as you might think since the floral nectars that comprise honey contain B vitamins and minerals which are calming to the nervous system.

Honegar

You can create a tonic stock that is stored at room temperature by combining 2 parts apple cider vinegar and 1 part honey. (Both are best purchased in the health food store for the most natural versions.) You need not refrigerate this stock, as honey is a natural preservative.

- ❀ When an emotional flare-up looks like it's about to hit, give 1 tablespoon of the Honegar stock mixed in ½ cup water, served either cold or hot as a tea.
- ❀ You can repeat this dosage several times a day if necessary.

TEEN ENERGY BOOSTERS

Typically, teens don't need much in the way of energy-boosting. But for the occasional doldrums or moments of dispiritedness, I like the following remedies:

Peppermint Bath

- ❀ Add 10 drops of peppermint to the morning bath to perk your teen (or, let's face it, yourself!) up.
- ❀ Your teenager can also drink peppermint tea infusions, a much healthier stimulant than coffee. With the popularity of coffee bars as the scene of social activity, caffeine intake has risen in teens . . . the very last thing the hyper, stressed body needs. Make your teen aware that coffee bars also sell herbal teas.

Siberian Ginseng

This stimulating tonic fortifies the body but doesn't provide the "rush" of other ginsengs. It helps increase stamina, especially in the presence of physical or mental stress, and thus is perfect for students. It is commonly used by athletes to promote endurance, and protects the body against environmental stress such as noise, fluorescent lighting, pollution, radiation, passive smoke, work, and emotional overloads . . . perfect for the student life! As an added benefit, this tonic strengthens and supports the endocrine system, especially the stress-sensitive adrenal glands.

* Give your teen 1 teaspoon diluted in an ounce of water or juice or put the dose in a cup of hot water to be had as a morning tea.
* A second dose can be taken, if needed, in the afternoon.

MOOD SWINGS

A teenager's mood swings are often due to hormonal flare-ups, high sugar intake, and/or stress. Stress so early in life? Certainly! This passage in life probably produces, in our ill-prepared adolescents, the most varied sources of stress they'll ever experience. Consider the pressure of school itself: major exams; deadlines; term papers; peer pressure; keeping up with fashion; after-school activities' demands on their time; sexual responsibilities; and, of course, life with their parents and siblings. Just thinking about all this makes me ever so grateful I don't have to repeat this time in my life!

Stress, be it physical (as in high sugar intake) or emotional, upsets the acid-alkaline balance (pH) of the body. A quick way to restore this balance is with the syrupy tonic called Honegar (see above).

St. John's Wort

Meditation, vigorous exercise, and a healthy diet are all good antidotes to mood swings. However, if your teenager is going through a particularly difficult time, the herb St. John's Wort could help see him through it. In my opinion, less is best, and the dosage can best be controlled by giving it in liquid extract form rather than in pre-measured capsules.

- ✿ Start with 10 drops in a little water, twice a day.
- ✿ If a larger dose is required, or if you'd rather provide more frequent doses, you can always increase this to 20–30 drops given two or three times a day. The smaller dose may be all that's needed to take the edge off, so your teenager can make better choices throughout the day.
- ✿ While physical dependency is not a problem with St. John's Wort, we can become emotionally dependent on any substance, even a natural one, so try not to continue the treatment for longer than a few months.

Bach Flower Essences

The emotional component of the teen years can be gently treated with Bach Flower Essences (see Appendix I for more on this). Impatience, scattered thinking, envy, depression, perfection, fear, low self-esteem, stubbornness . . . all are states of mind that can be subtly eased.

ACNE

Acne is best approached from the inside-out, as well as from the outside-in. I could never understand the age-old emphasis on skin cleansing as the cure-all for acne. Most teenagers suffering from acne are overly concerned with their appearance and the opinions of their peers, and spend more time cleaning their skin than any other humans on earth!

My teenaged clients find great improvements in their skin by using this three-tiered protocol:

1. The Outside-In Approach (topical cleansing and hydration with herbs)
2. Defining Food Intolerances
3. The Inside-Out Approach (internal cleansing of organs)

The Outside-In Approach

GENTLE FACIAL SCRUB

This approach includes exfoliation (sloughing of dead surface skin cells) using a facial scrub gentle enough to be used on a daily basis. Check your local health food store for a gentle, creamy scrub. My favorite scrub is handmade by a company called Gemma (see Appendix G for resource).

HONEY-NUTMEG CLEANSING MASK

This mask is great as a weekly treatment for deep pore cleansing, refining, and sloughing. It's easy to prepare and fun to use because the mask gets so sticky. You and your teen might like to do this one together . . . we sure did in my house.

- ❀ Combine 2 tablespoons honey with ½ to 1 teaspoon freshly grated nutmeg (depending upon how smooth or gritty you like it).
- ❀ Spread the mask on the face, keeping clear of eyes.
- ❀ Leave on 10 to 20 minutes.
- ❀ Before removing with warm water, press your fingers into the sticky mask and quickly pull away, to create a "tapping" sensation all over your face. This stimulates circulation and is fun to do with your teenager.

ALOE ACNE TREATMENT

Aloe is an excellent healing agent for the skin. Look for a cosmetic-quality aloe whipped with glycerine (see Appendix G for resources) to provide the healing and protective qualities of the plant as well as its anti-inflammatory, soothing, and hydrating properties. Apply morning and night as you would a moisturizer.

HERBAL ZINC ZAPPER

An excellent preparation to dry up new acne breakouts can be made in your kitchen.

- To a tube of zinc oxide cream add several drops oil of peppermint and just enough powdered comfrey to create a pleasing, spreadable consistency.
- Apply nightly or as needed.

HERBAL STEAMS

Aggravated skin can be cleansed and calmed with facial steams.

- To a pan of hot water, add 4–6 drops essential oils of geranium, chamomile, lavender, rosemary, or rose, or any combination of these oils that you especially like. (At fancy salons, customers are often asked to pick and choose among essential oils before a facial or massage. Why not concoct your own aromatherapeutic delight?)
- Cover your teen's head with a thick terrycloth towel and have her breathe in deeply, allowing the steam of the oils to penetrate the skin.
- A 5 to 10 minute steam will open the pores and allow the vapor of the anti-inflammatory, antimicrobial oils to be absorbed.
- Gently pat the skin dry and apply a soothing, anti-inflammatory, moisturizing botanical such as a cosmetic-quality aloe gel or chamomile cream.

The Inside-Out Approach

Junk foods leave a toxic waste in the body, as do stress hormones.

- An herbal detoxification program will help reduce toxic breakouts in the skin. (See Cleansing of the Internal Organs below.)
- Drinking 8 to 10 glasses a day of distilled water also helps flush toxic waste (as well as some minerals, so it's a good idea to add

a mineral supplement to the diet when one ingests large amounts of distilled water). Incidentally, based on the bio-rhythms of the body, minerals are best assimilated after 3 P.M., so be sure your teen takes the mineral supplements at night.

FOOD TESTING

Certain foods may not be well tolerated during adolescence. The first foods to consider should be sugar, wheat, and dairy. The offend-ing foods can be determined by kinesiological testing or through an elimination diet (see Appendix C for a discussion of both methods).

CONSTIPATION

Acne is often linked to constipation. A well-functioning colon will produce at least one or two easy bowel movements every day. Would you eat a piece of meat that had been sitting on a counter in sum-mer's heat for more than a day? Of course not. Similarly, matter retained in the colon at the normal body temperature of 98.6 degrees starts to putrefy, as would the meat. This produces an unnecessary burden on the body in the form of additional toxic by-products. When toxins cannot easily exit via the colon, they will exit through the largest eliminative organ in the body: the skin. Sufficient water and fiber must be included every day to ensure healthy, daily bowel movements.

CLEANSING OF THE INTERNAL ORGANS

Our beloved Dr. Christopher favored cleansing organs in concert rather than focusing on one organ at a time. Having used this approach myself for many years, I have found this to be a gentle yet effective way to detoxify the body.

When the kidneys, bladder, liver, bloodstream, and colon are functioning properly, they will help toxins exit the body efficiently. When there is an impediment to the proper evacuation of toxic mat-ter, often they will try to exit the body via the skin.

Following is a 4-week detoxification program that has helped many a teen cleanse internal organs and get them back on track when it comes to eating healthfully. The focus created by detoxing also helps teens focus on other aspects of their life that may need "cleansing."

Note: See Appendix H for the ingredients in these formulas so you can, if possible, find similar preparations in the health food store. If you wish to use these specific formulas, see Appendix G for resources.

As is true of all encapsulated herbs, it is important to drink lots of water when taking them. Remind your teen that these dried herbs were once plants that were full of water; they need to be rehydrated to be fully activated. Sometimes, when too little water is swallowed with the capsules, a bit of heartburn may be experienced. This is the body's signal that more water is required.

JUNI-PARS (KIDNEY AND BLADDER CLEANSER)

- *Dose*: two capsules three times a day, or three twice a day.
- Your teen will experience more frequent and/or fuller urinations, as these herbs stimulate the kidneys and bladder to cleanse toxic matter from the body.
- This formula is taken for the first two weeks of the cleansing period.

BARBERRY LG (LIVER AND GALLBLADDER CLEANSER)

- *Dose*: two to three capsules, 2–3 times a day for the full four week period. (Do less with the more petite child and more with the larger child.)
- The liver and gallbladder are fatty organs and, since fat retains toxins all too well, they require a longer, more focused time of cleansing.
- One of the liver's myriad functions is to process the chemicals to which we are exposed. After it is cleansed, it should be able to do its job better, thereby putting less burden on eliminative organs, such as the skin.

FEN LB (COLON CLEANSER)

- *Dose*: two capsules should be taken in the morning and two at bedtime.

♢ These herbs stimulate the colon, allowing it to cleanse itself of toxic residue.

♢ If your teen experiences diarrhea for more than three days, reduce the dose to one capsule or skip the morning dose.

♢ Take this formula for the full four weeks of the detox program to assist the toxins in exiting the body.

RED CLOVER COMBINATION (BLOOD CLEANSER)

♢ *Dose:* two capsules, 2–3 times a day.

♢ This formula will be taken for the last two weeks of the program. When Juni-Pars ends, start the Red Clover Combination.

♢ A concept helpful to understanding this formula's function is to picture it as the sweeper—sweeping out toxins that were stirred up but not yet released from the liver and bloodstream.

♢ It is important not to conclude detoxing before finishing the Red Clover Combination. Sometimes toxins can be experienced as symptoms of flulike headaches and achiness. Taking the Red Clover formula prevents this from occurring.

I cannot emphasize enough how important it is that your teen eat healthfully while doing this cleansing program. What would be the point of taking toxins out while pouring junk in? I don't think this will be a problem, however—because, as I mentioned above, the act of following a detoxification program usually encourages people (even teens!) to eat more healthfully.

Dr. Christopher's diet recommendation is for a "mucusless" diet consisting of grains, vegetables, fruits, nuts, seeds, and lots of water. Both his preference and mine is for distilled water.

COLON 8

If your teen suffers from constipation, I highly recommend doing a 10-day pre-detox cleansing of the colon with an herbal colon cleanser. A product I really like is Colon 8 (see Appendix H for ingredients, and Appendix G for resources). Colon 8 nourishes the colon as it cleanses. The rest of the detox will proceed more comfortably and effectively when this 10-day cleanse initiates the program.

MENSTRUAL CRAMPS

Gentle Ginger Compress

- ✿ Add two tablespoons fresh ginger root to 1½ cups water. Bring to a boil, reduce heat, and simmer for 20 minutes.
- ✿ Dip a cotton cloth into the hot liquid, remove with tongs or rubber gloves, and place over the area of discomfort. Waving the cloth mid-air for a moment or two will cool it enough to be comfortable on the skin.
- ✿ Cover with a hot water bottle to keep the compress warm.
- ✿ Keep in place for 20–30 minutes, repeating every couple of hours, if needed.

Dr. Christopher's Nu Fem Formula

If your teen's PMS is chronic and severe, symptoms may include (migraine) headaches, painfully swollen breasts, cramping, water retention, and/or mood swings. In this case, a deeper reproductive organ tonic/hormone balancer is required. Dr. John R. Christopher's Nu Fem formula is the best I've seen (see Appendix G for resources), dosed at two capsules three times a day for three months.

If your teen's periods need regulating because they are too heavy, too often, too late, or too light, giving the Nu Fem formula described above will help balance them.

I think my personal experience with this formula is probably worth telling, as it will help you to understand how very special this formula really is.

From the time I began menstruating at age 13, my periods were always sporadic, coming every 6, 8, 10, or 12 weeks. This condition continued well into my adult years. I certainly didn't mind having my period less often until I discovered I had difficulty conceiving. I wasn't ready to take the fertility drugs that my doctor was recommending and turned, instead, to the basal thermometer to try to determine when I was ovulating.

When I discovered I was only ovulating about once a year, I

knew that I really had to be diligent about charting my temperature, and that's how I conceived. Subsequently, the periods returned to their "normal" (that is to say, abnormal!) frequency. This didn't faze me until several years later when I was trying to conceive again. This time, my doctor recommended surgery; and again, I turned to the basal thermometer to chart my relatively infrequent ovulation. This method permitted me to conceive my second child.

Several years later, I began to face up to the fact that my menstrual cycle was anything but normal, and that this condition might be cause for difficulties later in life. I was living a healthy lifestyle and decided I should "walk the talk" and take charge of my hormonal imbalance. I took the Nu Fem formula just as described above for three months. My periods began to regulate, and started coming every 28 days; they have done so ever since, and I took this formula over 10 years ago. I never again took the Nu Fem formula. The herbs did their job by bringing the reproductive system into proper balance.

A TEEN TONIC

Raspberry leaf has long enjoyed a reputation as a "women's" herb because it has traditionally been used in many cultures throughout pregnancy as a strengthener of the uterus. However, raspberry leaf is also a marvelous all-around tonic for guys as well as gals in that it helps bolster the immune system and is also quite high in minerals. The addition of peppermint leaf makes this tonic a great replacement for coffee as a morning pick-me-upper. It's a tea the whole family can enjoy and is one of my personal favorites.

Raspberry Leaf Tonic Tea

   ☘ Steep 1 teaspoon raspberry leaf and ½ teaspoon peppermint leaf in one cup boiled water for 10–15 minutes (or more, if your teen likes a stronger flavor).

❀ Remember to cover the cup while steeping this tea to retain the lovely aromatic oils present in peppermint. Strain and serve.

❀ This tea may be had hot or cold on a daily basis, 2–3 times a day.

A book I highly recommend to the mothers of daughters for its refreshing and enlightened approach to the development of the female psyche is Dr. Joan Borysenko's *A Woman's Book of Life; The Biology, Psychology and Spirituality of the Feminine Life Cycle* (Riverhead Books, 1996).

ONE MORE THOUGHT . . .

My mother raised me with an oft-used expression: Have an educated heart. What she was trying to teach me was to think and act compassionately. In today's world, we put so much emphasis on intellect, scores, and goal attainment that our children often fail to receive adequate training for cultivating an educated heart. My mother, an early-childhood educator, has developed programs that teach loving values to children as young as two and three years old. Start early with your own children, and you will be giving them a gift that will enhance their communications and relationships throughout their lives.

The Institute of HeartMath, a nonprofit research and education organization in Boulder Creek, CA, teaches children that thinking with their hearts can enhance their health and ultimately reduce violence in schools. Using a method called Freeze-Frame, children are encouraged to step away from a stressful situation and recall positive feelings to counteract the damaging electrical impulses that race from the heart to the brain when they are angry or afraid. Children who use this technique restore balance to their hearts and brains, thereby bringing a positive emotional shift to a potentially explosive situation. Teens practicing conflict-resolution techniques such as "deep-heart listening" were found to have increased focusing skills and stronger peer empathy than those who did not have this training. Teaching young adults to get out of their heads and into their hearts is a way of nurturing emotional intelligence—or, as my mother so succinctly put it, having an educated heart.

For further reading about the Institute of HeartMath and its life-enhancing techniques, read Doc Lew Childre's book, *A Parenting Manual: Heart Hope for the Family* (Planetary Publications) or contact the Institute at 14700 West Park Avenue, Boulder Creek, CA 95006, Telephone: (831) 338-8700.

11

Calming the Jitters

Childhood today is, in many ways, more anxiety-provoking than when we were growing up. If we are indeed part of a global village, the upside is shared information and unlimited vistas; but that, along with pressures you and I never knew as kids, contributes to a world that is far more intense than the one I experienced, even as a girl in New York City!

To be sure, many of childhood's most troubling times are age-old issues. Being popular, pretty, handsome, smart, or athletic is hardly new, nor is that urgent need to somehow, some way "fit in." Yet the intense competition and striving for success that is the hallmark of today's world filters down to our youth more strongly than ever before.

Sadly, much of this is the result of expectations we have for our children from the day they are born. We all want our kids to do well, but must we plan their entry to elite kindergartens while they are still teething?

The result, of course, is a large number of kids who are always on edge. Sometimes this happens despite our best efforts as parents, and is the product of nature, not nurture. (In fact, New Yorker published an article in which a psychologist claimed that it is children's peer groups, more than the parents, that have the most marked affect on their personality, achievement, and inner lives.)

Happily, most kids outgrow the occasional jitters and are in fact happy campers most of the time. But I think you'll come to love, as I did, these nerve-calming herbal remedies that can restore equilibrium at even the rockiest of times.

HERBS TO CALM THE NERVOUS SYSTEM

Do consider the calming recommendations throughout this chapter. You may not be faced with an ADD/ADHD issue, for example, but there are many wonderful relaxing suggestions in that section.

What herbs are to the physical body, Bach Flower Essences are to the emotional body. Developed by English physician Dr. Edward Bach, the remedies promote wellness by addressing the mental and emotional counterparts to physical dysfunction, thus allowing a healthy life force to be released within the body/mind. The medical field of psychoneuroimmunology has clearly linked emotional conflict, such as fears, phobias, hate, anger, etc., to physical pathology.

The Essences, prepared vibrationally from flowers, contribute a subtle yet potent support for emotional reactions to emergency situations as in physical injury; the presence of long-term emotional challenges, as in sibling rivalry, a death in the family, or divorce; fears and phobias, and nightmares.

To make use of these wonderful substances, you can either follow the information detailed in the many books written on this subject or contact a practitioner in Bach Flower Essences, who can assist in developing a personalized formula specifically designed for your child.

Bach Flower Rescue Remedy

The Bach Flower Rescue Remedy can be used in any emergency situation, great or small. It is useful upon hearing sudden bad news, awaking from a nightmare, after an accident, prior to or postsurgery, or for pre-exam jitters. It addresses issues of shock, terror, panic, mental stress, tension, confusion, desperation, and even loss of consciousness. Rescue Remedy is meant to assist, not replace, appropriate medical treatment.

- Add 4 drops of Rescue Remedy (found at most health food stores) to a half glass of water, encouraging frequent sips.
- As your child grows calmer, decrease the frequency of sips.
- If the child is unable to sip or is unconscious, rub Rescue Remedy on the gums, lips, behind the ears, and on wrists at intervals as frequent as every five minutes until emergency medical help arrives.
- Several drops of Rescue Remedy can be applied directly to external injuries, used to bathe a painful area, or applied as a compress (6 drops to a pint of water).

I've even used it on our family pets! Our dog, April, was afraid of other neighborhood dogs, so I'd give this to her when her "friends" came to visit, with excellent results.

I will not tell you about the time our llamas escaped, and how half our town helped to track them down. But I will tell you that I gave Rescue Remedy to these "pets" by putting it in their water for heat stress on one especially hot summer day.

For more information, see Appendix I.

Tranquili-Tea

I created this formula to be used as a noncaffeinated, natural option for teatime. To me, teatime represents a period in the day to withdraw from the demands of the moment, to collect one's thoughts, and to get revitalized for the activities still ahead. (Or even to take a break from a day's shopping outing, which I consider most stressful of all!)

Children can also benefit from Tranquili-Tea's calming properties. Given in ¼ to ½ cup servings, it can bring relaxation to an overactive or overscheduled child during the day, or help him wind down in preparation for bedtime. It's a tea to benefit parent and child, especially when sipped together.

You can easily prepare a jar of this tea by combining the following herbs:

2 parts chamomile flowers
2 parts lemon balm leaves

½ part lemongrass
¼ part spearmint leaves (optional)

To prepare a cup of Tranquili-Tea:

- ❁ Pour a cup of boiled water over 1 teaspoon of the herbal combination.
- ❁ Steep, covered, 15 minutes. Strain before serving. Honey may be added to taste.

Spearmint is not considered a relaxing herb. The reason I have included it is to mask the taste of the chamomile. Imagine—an herbalist not in love with the taste of chamomile! Whenever I want to mask the flavor of an herb (for a child or for the adult with a child's palate), I add a little spearmint.

SLEEP PROBLEMS

Natural Approaches

Difficulties in getting to sleep or in staying asleep need to be addressed in several ways. The most obvious issue is to look at your child's nighttime activity preceding bedtime. In most homes, evening hours are filled with the hustle and bustle of dinner, homework, and sharing the day's happenings. All this is wonderful, but there's usually very little wind-down time, which in some cases may be all that's needed to normalize your child's sleep patterns. (After all, don't you give yourself some down time before retiring—with a little mindless TV or a good book?) Even your own pre-bed washing up or dental care can be relaxing for adults, whereas kids typically rush through this to get to the next activity or to get to bed "on time."

- ❁ Some relaxing yoga postures encourage deep breathing, and thus may be helpful.

☙ Similarly, easy imagery exercises can work wonders. Look for books devoted to these subjects to give you some ideas.

☙ For some children, certain foods need to be avoided before bedtime. Chief among these are sugary snacks or hard-to-digest foods like nuts. Experimentation will reveal which foods may prove problematic before bedtime.

☙ I have found that simply sharing quiet time with a warm cup of relaxing tea before bed, or even in bed, can provide not only wind-down time, but an intimate time of sharing for you and your child. This is also an excellent time to release concerns and fears he may have. In the health food store, you can find relaxing herbal teas designed for children, or try my personal favorite:

Peaceful Dreams Tea

☙ Combine 1 teaspoon chamomile flowers, 1 teaspoon lemon balm leaf, and ¼ teaspoon spearmint leaf.

☙ Pour 1½ cups boiled water over the herbs, cover the cup, and allow to steep for 10–20 minutes.

☙ Strain and serve half to each of you. You can add a bit of honey as a sweetener, if you like.

Essential Oils

☙ To make the night-light that children often sleep with a healing tool, purchase an electric (not candle) aromatherapy lamp. (This can usually be found in stores selling natural products.) The heat of this low-wattage light can diffuse a scent that is relaxing to the nervous system; the essential oils of lavender and chamomile are among the very best. Follow the directions provided with the lamp as to quantities of oil that should be used.

☙ Little sleep pillows can be purchased or made. Relaxing herbs and essential oils are enclosed in the pillows and can be placed next to your child's head.

☙ If your child sleeps with a favorite stuffed animal, you can tuck a piece of cloth doused with essential oils inside its body. Do this by creating an opening in its seam and adding a snap so the scented cloth can be renewed when the aroma fades.

Herbal Extracts

Health food stores offer sleep-enhancing formulas designed especially for children. All of these herbs are classified as nervines, which are soothing to the nervous system. These formulas usually contain a combination of: valerian root, skullcap, hops, passionflower, chamomile, oats.

NAIL BITING

Generally, nail biting is a nervous response, so the first herbs to look to are the nervines, discussed above.

Topical Deterrents

Another way to approach nail biting is to create a "flagging system."
- ✿ Gently tie something fun to the fingers as a reminder not to bite the nails. Brightly colored strips of cloth work well.
- ✿ Even better, have your child become a part of the deterrent process by coloring the strips of cloth with nontoxic coloring pens.
- ✿ Cloth-covered elastic hair ties can also work.
- ✿ Finger cots (old-fashioned rubberized covers for fingers designed to help turn pages more easily and available in stationery stores) can be decorated to look like funny faces and placed over the favorite nail-biting fingers.

FEARS AND ANXIETIES

The suggestions for helping your child get to sleep also apply to easing fears and anxieties. If more herbal help is needed, consider:

- Bach Flower Essences. Dr. Bach's flower essences are to the emotions what herbs are to the body. Children are very responsive to their gentle energetic properties. See Appendix I for further description.
- *Kali Phos.* This is a cell salt (see Appendix F for discussion of cell salts) that nourishes and relaxes the nervous system. For the child with a jittery disposition, you may use this on an ongoing basis.

ATTENTION DEFICIT DISORDER (ADD)
ATTENTION DEFICIT HYPERACTIVE DISORDER (ADHD)

The debate on attention deficit disorders is among the most raging concerns of educators, physicians, and parents alike. In fact, entire books have been written about the subject, so I won't attempt to present a comprehensive review of the disorder's etiology, especially since the causational factors range from sociological to ecological to biological—and to many minds, the jury is still out on this paradoxical condition.

Similarly, there are no hard-and-fast solutions that apply to all children. Indeed, in *Time* Magazine (November 30, 1998), an article entitled "The Age of Ritalin" discusses the fact that in just one year, doctors wrote half a million Ritalin prescriptions for 3-to-6-year-olds in this country alone. That said, no one in the medical or psychiatric communities is absolutely certain that ADD and ADHD are, in fact, neurochemical imbalances; thus, medication may not be the best way to treat these disorders. Further, there are no long-term studies on the extended use of this medication. In the same vein, many children suffering from depression are being treated with antidepressant drugs, even though the FDA has not approved their use for children under the age of 18.

I have found that for virtually all my ADD and ADHD clients, the use of herbs, coupled with dietary changes, have helped these children function much better both at home and in school. Some of these children have even been able to avoid the use of prescribed pharmaceuticals; others have had their doses reduced; and others still have been able to come off the drugs after implementing suggested changes.

Diet

I firmly believe that much of ADD and ADHD is the result of undiagnosed food allergies and sensitivities. When children ingest these offending foods, they become irritable and emotionally reactive because the foods act as irritants to the nervous system. Sugar is a primary offender, as are food dyes, fast foods, prepackaged foods, and any foodstuff containing additives, preservatives, MSG, sulfites, and other hidden chemicals.

You can discover your child's food sensitivities by using kinesiology, described in Appendix C. As I discuss there, the most frequent offenders are wheat, dairy, corn, peanuts, and chocolate. Rather than eliminating all possible offenders, kinesiology, also known as energy testing or muscle testing, will help you specifically define those foods that present a problem to your child.

To ascertain the effect that food is having, test every food ingested, and eliminate everything that doesn't test well for one week; be sure to keep a diary of behavioral responses. You may find that a certain food group is best replaced by another; e.g., rice products can replace those made with wheat (like pasta and bread), or soy for dairy (as in soy milk, soy cheese, and soy-based ice cream).

Sometimes the way a food is processed is the key to the sensitivity your child experiences. In fact, one brand may "test" better than another. Never guess or assume; test everything, even vitamins, which may seem harmless because they are "natural," but which may be loaded with sugars and dyes. Check the label in every case.

If food sensitivities are not the root cause of ADD/ADHD, you should still eliminate the offenders from your child's diet. By eliminating the dietary challenges to your child's immune system, a more comfortable level of functioning may be experienced.

Herbs

I advise using the following herbs in liquid-extract form because you can mix together small amounts of any or all of them to create a formula most beneficial to your child's individual needs. Using the guidelines in the chapter on dosing, keep adjusting and observing until the right mix is attained. You must be vigilant, because it is possible that a different combination will best serve your child in the morning and another at bedtime. For help in developing a formula for your child, see page 183.

- St. John's Wort helps relieve anxiety and mild depression.
- Ginkgo increases the child's ability to focus by increasing circulation to the cerebral vascular system.

Nervines are a classification of herbs that calm and nourish the nervous system. They are also helpful in counteracting the sleep problems that often accompany ADD/ADHD drug therapy; they are nonaddictive and have a long, rich history of use. Nervines include:

- Passionflower, which helps sleep disturbances, and helps reduce anxiety and irritability. Its relaxing and antispasmodic properties also help reduce nervous hyperactivity and help improve concentration.
- Valerian root. The less common varieties of valerian have been found to help children with learning challenges because these herbs improve concentration and reduce anxious behavior.
- German chamomile flowers or Roman chamomile are soothing to the nerves, calm the digestive system; they also reduce irritability, muscle tension, and sleeping problems.

❀ Lemon balm helps to reduce nervous irritability and improve sleep.

❀ Gotu Kola has been shown to enhance attention span and concentration.

HOW TO TAILOR A FORMULA TO YOUR CHILD

❀ First determine which symptoms need to be addressed.

❀ Select the herb or herbs mentioned above that apply.

❀ Using the dosing guidelines in Chapter 3, determine the total amount of drops your child would require in a dose.

❀ Using your judgment about what to use more or less of, combine the liquid herbs to equal the total amount of the required dose.

❀ When giving the dose to your child, dilute it in an ounce or two of water or juice.

❀ You may wish to make up about three day's worth of the formula you have designed so that it doesn't have to be newly created for every dose. Eventually, when you have arrived at the best combination, you may wish to make up a supply that will last a month or two.

❀ Observe your child's response to the formula you have created. Make detailed notes regarding the exact ingredients of the formula used and resulting behavior. Adjust the formula as needed until you and your child are comfortable with its action.

❀ Keep in mind you may wish to create two separate formulas: one for daytime activities and another for sleep.

Essential Fatty Acids

Essential fatty acids (EFAs) are what we call "good fats" and can be extremely nourishing to the nervous system. Children with ADD/ADHD have shown improved concentration, reduction in hyperactivity, and a calmer constitution when EFAs, particularly fish oils, are added to their diet. A visit to your health food store will supply you with just the right product.

Essential Oils

The essential oil of a plant is its most potent component, and can be inhaled for aromatherapeutic effects. For their calming properties, the essential oils of lavender, chamomile, lemon, orange, tangerine, or rose can be:

- ❀ Heated in an aromalamp
- ❀ Added to a bath
- ❀ Used to scent a pillowcase
- ❀ Diluted in a vegetable or nut oil, and massaged into the skin. (A few drops to a teaspoon of a mild oil such as almond or sunflower is best.)

AROMATIC MASSAGE OIL

Create a calming, pleasant-smelling blend of 10 drops essential oils (see choices mentioned above) and combine with 1 ounce unscented vegetable or nut oil (almond, sunflower, apricot kernel, grapeseed). Massage the blended oil into the soles of the feet before nap or bedtime.

AROMALAMP

Add 10 drops of the aromatic massage oil to an ounce of water in the reservoir of an electric aromalamp. The gentle light and scent of the lamp infuses the child's bedroom with a quieting energy.

SCENTED PILLOW

Lightly douse a cotton handkerchief with several drops of the calming essential oils noted above, and slip inside your child's pillowcase.

AROMATIC BATH

- ❀ Add 10 drops of the aromatic massage oil to your child's bath water.
- ❀ Teach her how to derive the most benefit from this therapeutic form of hydrotherapy by closing her eyes and breathing deeply and slowly.

❀ The addition of quiet, soothing music can make bath time a calming therapy just before bedtime.

Vitamins and Minerals

Consult with a nutritionist to be sure your child is receiving proper supplementation. Nervous disorders can result from insufficient nutrition.

Calcium and magnesium are minerals that calm the nervous system. The herbs oatstraw and horsetail contain an easily assimilated form of these minerals. Children can enjoy the herbs in a drink I call Bone Tea Punch (so named because the minerals are also good for strengthening bones).

BONE TEA PUNCH

To prepare a large quantity of the dried herb mixture, combine and store in an air-tight container:

½ cup horsetail
½ cup oatstraw
½ cup chamomile

❀ Steep 3 teaspoons of the herb mixture in 3 cups boiled water until cooled.
❀ Add 1 cup of a favorite juice and chill.
❀ The fun part of Bone Tea Punch is that you can keep the flavor interesting by changing the kind of juice you add.

The same herb mixture can be used to make a relaxing bedtime tea.

❀ Pour 1 cup boiled water over 1 teaspoon of the dried herb mixture and steep for 15 minutes.
❀ A little honey may be added to sweeten.

Chemicals in Your Child's Home and School Environment

As you would foods, muscle test substances to keep sensitivity challenges to a minimum. (See Appendix C.) At home, test detergents, body soaps, lotions, and hair products. Refrain from using sprays and fragrances of all kinds.

Try to keep your home as dust-free as possible, removing stuffed animals from the child's immediate vicinity. Be sure to wash new linens and clothing before use.

In the daycare or school environment, test art supplies, including markers, chalk, glue, and cleaning products.

Empower Your Child!

Encourage her to participate in the selection and preparation of health-promoting foods. Whether at home or in the supermarket, make food-testing sessions fun and informative by pointing out how a certain food weakens or strengthens her. Whenever possible, help her to observe how she feels (good or bad) after ingesting particular foods.

Your child cannot help but feel deprived when others are delighting in cupcakes, ice cream, candy, and soda. Party time can therefore be particularly distressing; allow your child to choose substitute foods to bring to the party. Supply extra so she can share her goodies with others.

One Last Thought . . .

Have your child checked for candida. The inability to focus, behavioral problems, and sugar/food sensitivities can all be symptoms of this yeast-related health concern.

THE HEALING POWER OF MUSIC

Approximately 70 colleges in the U.S. offer degree programs in music therapy. Many health insurance programs consider music therapy a reimbursable health expense.

Far more than just a tool to soothe the anxious spirit, research has shown that music can impact brain development and cognitive functioning. It has the power to relax tense muscles by triggering physiological cellular responses.

Immune function has been shown to improve significantly with vocalization, such as singing or chanting. The use of music in biofeedback training has helped reduce migraines. Music therapy has reduced the incidence of seizures, and has improved concentration in children who have attention deficit disorders.

"Music is the most complementary medicine of the future," writes Dr. Don Campbell in *The Mozart Effect* (Avon, 1997). "When we are out of harmony, music can reorchestrate our lives for the health of mind, body, and soul." Campbell has developed a series of compact discs for children, "The Mozart Effect for Kids" (The Children's Group), in which he harnesses the power of tones, rhythms, and sounds to influence mental performance, spiritual outlook, and disease. For more information on Campbell and his fascinating research, you can log on to his Web site at www. Mozarteffect.com.

To help my sons shed the stresses of the day and allow them to fall asleep more easily, I gave them tapes containing meditations and classical music. If music can enhance concentration and focus, play Mozart softly in the background while your child does homework. It is also an excellent idea to stimulate your child's immune system with music while recuperating from illness.

We all recognize how music can negatively impact our children. Why not use its many positive attributes to help heal our youth?

A Word on Mindful Living . . .

There was a time when being a child meant having the time to lose one's self in a book, listen to records over and over, play alone with trucks, dolls, building blocks, or stuffed animals. These were times in which children focused on the one activity of the moment, activities that exercised the imagination. Without putting a name to it, these were opportunities for meditative play.

No Time to Think. All too often, today's child is ushered from one activity to the next. Play dates, music lessons, sports, homework, dance lessons—honestly, I feel that some parents measure their own worth by the number of activities their children are signed up for, or as if they were already plotting what to put on college applications!

For most children, there aren't that many hours between the end of extracurricular activities and bedtime. Free time, what there is of it, is spent with television and computer games. And for working parents, time to share is sandwiched in between dinner and bedtime. Where is the time for meditative, nonrushed activity? Where is the time to be alone, to let one's thoughts take wing?

When we adults drive, if we keep the radio, cassette, or CD player turned off, we have time to think. I do my best thinking when I drive. When we chauffeur our children, we use that precious time alone with them to "communicate." No time for meditative thought there!

The Path to Stress-Related Illness. Statistics reveal that cardiovascular disease is the #1 killer and costs the United States more than $150 billion every year. Approximately 150 million people are suffering from stress-related, chronic illness. The cost of running health care in this country is expected to reach $2 trillion by the year 2000. Many of our children are already experiencing stress-related syndromes that manifest in their psychological and physical health.

Does this have to be the future of the health of our children? Let's stop cramming so much into their lives, as if this were their last day on Earth. If this indeed were their last day, wouldn't it be better to fill it with loving expression, deep breaths of joy, and communication with their own souls to carry them into the hereafter? Some beautiful music wouldn't hurt either! How about incorporating these acts into their daily lives, even once a week? I believe the best way to make this happen is to look at our own lives first.

Enjoying the Moment. By teaching our children how to meditate, live mindfully, and not to run from one activity to the next while they are still young, we will be teaching them how to manage stress. What a great lesson in prevention this is. Certainly, we don't have to bog children down with the details of how to avoid heart attacks, diabetes, colitis, ulcers, hypertension, or back problems. Rather, just teach them the positives: how to eat and live mindfully and healthfully. Doesn't that sound simple? It really is, you know. Time and time again, my sons have pulled me up short, reminding me to be in the moment. At times, I would be so focused on the next activity that I would lose the enjoyment of the one I was in with them. That, my friends, is a real breath-prompter—when your own children see you stressed out, not practicing what you've shared with them over the years. (Thanks, guys: I take your lessons to heart—literally!)

If you need some help reconnecting yourself, check out the many wonderful books and recordings available in the library, bookstores, and on the Internet.

Immune System Enhancers

May the Force Be with You. The expression "to heal" shares the same Greek derivation as the phrase "to be whole." To be whole is to be balanced in one's spiritual life; in how we think and express ourselves; and in our bodily functions. We cannot *acquire* the power to heal ourselves, for it is a power that dwells within us. The force that drives the brilliant communication among our cells is ready to fully express itself at all times if we so allow it. How we think, eat, and live our lives can support or hinder the expression of our health and wholeness. When illness is the manifestation of our unbalanced lifestyles, herbal medicine and other natural therapies are tools that can be helpful in restoring this balance.

The Holistic Approach. Conventional medicine's approach to the immune system is to aggressively attack our body's attackers with an arsenal of synthetic compounds, thereby suppressing symptoms. However, this approach fails to address why the body was receptive to the invasion in the first place. Also, it is not always beneficial to do the dirty work for the body, but rather to help the body do the job it was designed to do.

Viewing the body holistically, as an integrated whole, rather than mechanically, as malfunctioning parts needing repair, provides us with an opportunity to understand why a body was originally receptive to microbial attack. Holistic medicine's approach, stimulating the body's own forces into action, facilitates the body's return to its natural state of balance.

Complementing Antibiotic Therapy. If a raging infection attacks a child's weakened immune system—a system too weak to successfully fight back—you may choose to use an antibiotic. However, after the antibiotic therapy is completed, the child's system will be no stronger than before the infection's attack.

This would be an excellent time to strengthen the immune system to help create a strong constitution. One way is to replenish the intestinal tract with plenty of probiotics (live bacterial microorganisms that naturally live in the intestinal tract and are responsible for keeping harmful organisms in check).

Natural yogurt contains acidophilus, a probiotic culture, and can be given to your child with a little fruit or a drizzle of honey.

Supplements of acidophilus can be given during the antibiotic therapy—and for a few weeks after its completion, to repopulate the intestinal tract with the "good guys." Give acidophilus 3 times a day, keeping it an hour away from the antibiotic.

Giving the last dose just before bedtime helps promote unimpeded multiplication of the "good guys" overnight. By supporting the growth of good bacteria, the immune system will be enhanced.

Lay a Healthy Foundation. What you don't give your child is just as important as what you do give to help build a stronger body. Not giving sugar-laden, chemical-laced foods would be most wise. This is also a fine time to test for food sensitivities (see Appendix C on food testing) so as to eliminate any foods that may not be strengthening the body's energy field. A diet based on small amounts of lean meat, poultry, fish and eggs, grains, seeds, nuts, fruits, and vegetables (organic, when possible) and lots of purified water will help lay a healthy foundation.

My children were not denied an occasional soft drink outside the home, but the drink of choice was water or water diluted with a little fruit juice for flavor. Milk was never drunk by the glassful, but in small amounts in cereal. Often soymilk was used in cereal or shakes.

Our bodies are constantly exposed to disease-producing organisms, namely viruses, parasites, bacteria, fungi; this is part of life. In strengthening your child's constitution with health-promoting foods and exercise, your child's body will maintain a vigorous level of self-protection and not fall prey to life's daily challenges. And, when occasionally he does, he will get well faster and his body's vitality will quickly be restored.

Foods to Support the Immune System

There are many opportunities for giving your children healthful, immune-enhancing foods in their daily diets.

However, if your child is a highly selective eater, consulting with a nutritionist can teach you how best to supplement her diet with health-promoting substances she may not be getting from her regularly eaten foods. This not only benefits your child's health, but helps contribute to your own peace of mind!

The following food suggestions contribute to the health of the immune system by cleansing and nourishing the body, as well as stimulating those important disease-fighting cells. Rather than concentrating on making a focused therapy of one of them, try to develop an ease about incorporating a variety of health-promoting supports in your family's diet.

- Red clover blossoms, fresh or dried, can be made into a hot or iced tea drink or the tea can be frozen into ice pops. A punch could be made from red clover tea and a favorite fruit juice.
- Dandelion greens can be added raw to a salad or steamed with other greens.
- A fun springtime family activity is identifying the health-promoting "weeds" growing in your lawn and picking them (if not chemically treated) for use in salads. Chickweed, red clover, plantain, and dandelion leaves are "noxious" weeds

people look to chemically eliminate from their lawns. At our house, we preferred to eliminate these healthful herbs by eating them!

- ✿ Garlic can be finely minced and served on buttered toast or added to mashed potatoes.
- ✿ Lemons, water and honey can be made into a hot cleansing morning lemonade or chilled for a refreshing cold drink.
- ✿ Burdock root can be served as a vegetable, thinly sliced and steamed or stir-fried, or as a tea.
- ✿ Beets can be grated and served raw over salads, juiced with other vegetables, steamed with potatoes, or made into a soup.
- ✿ Onions can be added raw or steamed to prepared foods. Steamed or stir-fried with honey, they make a delicious vegetable on their own.
- ✿ Flaxseeds can be sprinkled on cereal to promote healthy function of the colon.

Fresh Nettles

If you have the chance to harvest fresh nettles, you can lightly steam them for a highly nutritious vegetable. But beware: nettles, also known as stinging nettles, have sharp hairs on their leaves' undersides to protect the plant from natural prey. So how do you pick stinging nettles? As the old joke goes . . . very carefully! To avoid getting a nettles rash, I use spaghetti tongs. Once steamed, the nettles' sharp hairs magically disappear and you are left with a tender, delicious vegetable. This is a unique herb, indeed.

Mineral Tonic Tea

Nettle leaf and raspberry leaf are herbs that are high in minerals and great as nourishing tonics. If your kids won't eat their vegetables, perhaps they'll drink them. This is an excellent daily tonic for nursing mothers as well, since the herbs also serve to enhance the production of milk.

In this formula, the addition of spearmint gives nettles' "grassy" flavor a refreshing minty taste. Combine:

1 teaspoon nettles leaf
½ teaspoon raspberry leaf
½ teaspoon spearmint leaf

* Pour one cup boiled water over herbs; cover cup; steep 15 minutes.
* Strain and offer in ½ cup servings, warm or iced; sweeten with honey to desired taste.
* If you are giving this tea to your child as a daily tonic, you can prepare a larger quantity and store the tea in the refrigerator for up to three days.
* You can freeze the tea into ice pops. This is a good way to be sure your picky eater is taking in some daily nutrients.

Immune-Boosting Soup

An easy way to get your youngsters to eat more nutritiously is by putting medicinal herbs and health-promoting vegetables into a delicious soup.

* In a large cooking pot half-filled with water, simmer until softened any combination of: cruciferous, antioxidant-rich vegetables (broccoli, cauliflower, cabbage); carrots; leafy greens (kale, collards, mustard greens, turnip greens, dandelion greens, beet greens, spinach); shiitake mushrooms; onions; garlic; ginger; cayenne pepper (just a little, to stimulate circulation); burdock root; astragalus root (which can be purchased in most Asian markets).
* If your child prefers pureed soups, you can remove the mushrooms and roots after simmering; then puree to a thick, smooth soup.

EXCELLENT ALL-AROUND IMMUNE ENHANCERS

Siberian Ginseng

Known as a tonic herb, Siberian ginseng—note that this is different from other ginsengs—protects the body against stress; endogenous stress (from within the body such as emotional or chronic physical challenges), and external stress factors such as environmental pollutants. Siberian ginseng gives nourishment to the adrenal glands, which are highly reactive to stress. If your child could use a morning boost, try starting his day off with this wonderful immune-enhancing herb in the form of a tea, liquid extract, or capsule. See Chapter 3 for dosing guidelines.

Echinacea

Parents of my school-aged clients use echinacea to help keep their children healthy by giving them doses twice a day during the school week. It is especially beneficial to children entering a daycare, nursery, or kindergarten setting, where exposure to other children's germs occurs on a daily basis. In my home, we use echinacea preventatively throughout flu season.

You may wish to consider using echinacea when long-term emotional upset begins affecting the immune system. Six-year-old Michael found the school setting to be a supportive, loving environment—in contrast, unfortunately, with his home life on the weekends. His parents were in counseling in an attempt to save their marriage, and when everyone was home on the weekend, the tension was emotionally and physically challenging to Michael. He would respond with frequent upper respiratory infections, which flared up during or just after the weekends.

It didn't take too long for his parents to realize that the family stress was taking its toll on Michael's immune system. They began dosing him with echinacea on Friday to Sunday; this therapy helped him stay strong for his return to school on Monday. It was a good preventative application of echinacea's immune-enhancing properties.

Echinacea is an herb that has transformed more families' lives than

any other herb I know. It is also the most misused herb. To understand why, a brief and simple lesson in pharmacology will help.

IN WHAT FORM TO USE ECHINACEA

Some herbs are water-soluble, some are alcohol-soluble, and others
are both water- and alcohol-soluble. The solubility factor of an herb
is what helps determine how its chemical constituents are extracted.
Peppermint leaf is an example of a water-soluble herb. If you steep
peppermint in a cup of boiled water, its healing agents will be drawn
out and into that cup of water. Osha root, on the other hand, is
100% alcohol-soluble. Put osha root in a cup of boiled water and
you will get . . . nothing! It must be prepared in an alcohol base.

Let's return to the herb under discussion, echinacea, which is
both water- and alcohol-soluble. Echinacea needs both mediums
to extract all of its healing constituents. A liquid extract, prepared
with alcohol and water, therefore, is the most effective way to take
echinacea.

I know, I know: you're raising your eyebrows because I'm suggesting you give an alcohol preparation to your child. Well, if I want the
most from this wondrous herb, that's exactly what I do. Alcohol
extracts are given even to infants. An infant's dose is only a few
diluted drops, so the alcohol content is minuscule. If you want to get
rid of the alcohol, simply put the dose in hot water for a minute. In
my family, and in my clients' families, the same bottle of echinacea,
in liquid extract form, is used for both adults and children alike.

WHY AND HOW TO USE ECHINACEA

While echinacea does have antibacterial and antiviral properties, its
hallmark activity is in stimulating the immune system by charging
up those helper T-cells and killer T-cells.

- ❧ At the first sign of illness, begin with a full dose, always dilut-
  ing the dose in an ounce or two of juice or water. This could
  be a tickle in your child's throat, glassy eyes, or whatever is
  your child's first signal of "something coming."
- ❧ Give ½ dose every 2 hours until the symptoms have disappeared. If you've caught it quickly, only a few doses may be

necessary. This is why I travel with a small dropper bottle of echinacea wherever I go, so dosing can begin before anything significant develops.

✿ If it's gotten a foothold in your child's system, repeat the ½ dose every two hours for a day or so (until your child feels better).

✿ Then give a full dose three times a day until completely well, for up to 10 days.

HOW TO DOSE A CHILD WITH ECHINACEA

✿ An adult's full dose of echinacea is 1 teaspoon.

✿ The simple formula for dosing a child is to use an adult weight of 150 pounds to be divided by the child's weight. If the child weighs 50 pounds, then dividing 150 by 50 would mean that the child should receive ⅓ the adult dose, or ⅓ teaspoon diluted in a little water or juice.

✿ Because children of the same age can vary greatly in size, always use your child's weight to determine the correct dose.

Why stop giving echinacea at 10 days? Why is more not always better? Echinacea is a safe, nontoxic herb. However, studies reveal that its efficacy peaks at ten days and then wanes. In order not to lose its effectiveness, it is best to stay on it through the peaking period, come off for a few days, and then, if required, resume taking it to get another boost to the immune system.

The only caveat that I am aware of with echinacea is in cases of autoimmune disease. The studies are not conclusive as to whether echinacea could aggravate rather than help in these situations, so to be on the safe side, I would recommend against its use if your child has an autoimmune disease until more information is available.

WHEN TO GIVE ECHINACEA

Ongoing therapy with echinacea is effective for people who find stress an immunodepressant. Stress can come in many forms. What stresses one individual means nothing to another. Stress can be emotional, physical, or environmental. Flu season, for example, is stressful. It is important to teach your child ways of handling stress, and to help support your child's body when it is going through periods of prolonged stress.

- ✿ When my children were little, I'd ask them to tell me what was going on in school around them, healthwise. If other kids were dropping like flies, we'd go on repeated rounds of echinacea— 10 days on, then 4 days off, especially during November to April's flu season. We never had flu or any other illness rampage through our household, because we knew how to protect ourselves.
- ✿ If other children in your child's daycare setting are sick, it would be a good idea to put your child on echinacea during the week and off it for the weekend.
- ✿ If your child is sublimely happy during the school week but finds life at home on the weekends difficult (perhaps, like Michael, due to a trying family situation), then taking echinacea from Friday to Sunday may be the best plan.
- ✿ If your child does take ill, give ½ dose of echinacea every two hours and give a full dose to siblings and parents three times a day until the sick child is well. By doing so, you protect the whole family.
- ✿ If a child comes home from a play date and says that the friend was coming down with a cold, protect your child with echinacea. Because it is such a safe herb, I have always "erred" on the side of giving it to my children—or taking it myself!— rather than not.

By the way, echinacea doesn't taste real good, so you might want to give the dose in a bit of juice. My sons were brought up with the notion that shot glasses were designed for herbs, because that's how they always were given their doses of echinacea. They went off to college with their very own shot glasses, still using them (as I do) for doses of liquid extracts. My youngest began college with two full bottles of echinacea, which he quickly exhausted. Concerned that he was ill, I asked why he needed replenishment so quickly. Brian explained that everyone in his dorm was sick, and he was taking the herb to protect himself. (Of course, he also offered it to anyone who would take it!) Start your kids off with the understanding that they can do something wonderful to keep themselves healthy, and they will carry this proactive preventive knowledge with them for the rest of their lives.

FEVER-FIGHTING HERBS

A fever is the body's way of letting you know there's an infection present, and that your child's army of defenses is engaged in battle. While it is not good to let the fever get out of control because of the dangerous effects it can have on the body, it is also not good to immediately suppress it. Parents new to natural healing therapies usually call upon aspirin substitutes when the temperature rises above 103 degrees, and safely use herbal therapies for reducing temperatures below 103. As you become more confident with the tools available from nature's pharmacy, you will become less reliant upon conventional medicine and drug therapy.

Get a Medical Diagnosis

It is important to have a persistent fever medically diagnosed. Its source can be as simple as a cold, or it can be something far more serious that may require medical attention. Herbal therapies can be given in conjunction with conventional medicine, but you need to know for certain what it is you are dealing with. Get a medical opinion, make your educated decision, and then discuss with your child's pediatrician the direction you plan on taking.

Herbal Baths

You can immerse your child into a warm herbal bath, give him a sponge bath, or simply compress affected areas of the body to help cool it down. Afterward, be sure to keep your child warm and covered with a blanket until the fever reduces.

- ❀ Prepare a quart infusion of chamomile, peppermint, elderflower, or lavender—or any combination of these diaphoretic teas. (See Appendix A for preparation guidelines.) Their chemical properties encourage sweating, a function that helps cool down the body as well as release toxins.
- ❀ The quart infusion may be added to bath water.
- ❀ It may be used to sponge bathe the child.
- ❀ A compress may be made by dipping a cotton cloth into the infusion and holding it against the head, neck, chest, stomach, and feet.
- ❀ If your child develops the chills after the bath or compresses, ginger tea (see Appendix A for preparing a decoction) diluted with half as much pineapple juice will help build circulation and warm the body.
- ❀ It is very important to keep your child well hydrated with teas, water, and diluted juices during this time.

Herbal Teas

The purpose of these teas is to encourage perspiration, allowing toxins to release through the skin and cool the body. Be sure to keep your child warm and covered with a blanket until the fever reduces.

- ❀ Begin by giving 1–2 droppersful of yarrow or elderflower tea every 10–15 minutes for the first hour.
- ❀ Increase dose to ¼ to ½ cup tea, while reducing frequency to every ½ hour for an hour or two.
- ❀ Maintain dose, but reduce frequency to every hour for two hours, then every few hours, until the fever reduces.
- ❀ The teas may be continued 3 or 4 times a day for a few days to support the immune system.
- ❀ If there is chest involvement, a teaspoon of sage or mullein

may be steeped with a teaspoon of yarrow or elderflower in 1½ cups water for 15–30 minutes.

Herbs to Bolster the Immune System

In addition to the above teas, support the immune system with the following herbs (also see Chapter 5 for more detail on giving echinacea and garlic):

- ⚜ Echinacea extract diluted in a little juice every 2 hours (giving a dose of vitamin C with every dose of echinacea will enhance its action).
- ⚜ Garlic oil, perles, tablets, or a fresh, chopped clove in food every few hours.
- ⚜ Goldenseal capsules or extract diluted in a little juice can be given 3 to 4 times a day. *Note:* Do not buy the combined echinacea/goldenseal extract, as you will want to give the former more frequently than the latter.
- ⚜ For a fever that is not responding to aspirin substitutes or herbal therapies, see the garlic fever reducer in Chapter 6.
- ⚜ Aspirin is to be avoided as it has the potential to cause Reye's Disease in children.

Vaporizing Herbs

- ⚜ Several drops of antimicrobial essential oils of eucalyptus, tea tree, thyme, lemon, or lavender can be added to a vaporizer to be dispersed in the air in your child's room.
- ⚜ If your child is suffering from congestion, you can make a steam tent of the essential oil of eucalyptus for the nasal passages or thyme for the chest (or a combination of both, if needed) by putting 2–4 drops (total) into a pan of hot water. Cover his head and the pan with a terrycloth towel and have him inhale the steam from the herbal water for 5 to 10 minutes.

❀ See Chapter 5 on the Upper Respiratory System for a formula for Head-Clearing Tea and other decongesting herbal remedies.

Cell Salts for Fever

The Biochemic Handbook (Chapman & Perry [revised 1994]), a repertory for cell salts, lists the following cell salts for specific symptoms accompanying fever:

Ferr. Phos. The principal remedy for high temperatures, quickened pulse, and feverishness.

Kali Sulph. In alternation with Ferr. Phos., to control the temperature and to promote perspiration.

Kali Phos. Nervous fevers, high temperature, quick and irregular pulse with general nervous excitement.

Kali Mur. Catarrhal fevers, great chilliness, with white-coated tongue and constipation.

Nat. Mur. Hay fever with watery discharge; dryness of the bowel or other symptoms pointing to a disturbance in the moisture regulating process.

Nervine Herbs

If the fever is causing achiness and difficulty sleeping, giving a nervine formula a few times a day, or only in the evening, will help to relax the muscles and promote sleep. Valerian, passionflower, hops, and skullcap are examples of herbs that relax and nourish the nervous system. Look for a formula of nervine herbs in your local health food store.

Bach Flower Remedies

A child may become fearful or fretful with a fever. See Appendix I on Bach Flower Essences for help with emotional issues related to the illness.

ALLERGIES

An allergy is the body's exaggerated response to a substance its immune modulators find offensive. Allergic responses manifest in a variety of ways. Severe anaphylactic reactions (e.g., closing of throat, elevated pulse, shock) are life-threatening and require immediate emergency treatment. The more common allergic response can be experienced as discomforts of the skin, including hives, rashes, eczema; or of the respiratory system: runny nose, nasal congestion, itchy eyes, headaches, coughs, and asthma are the most frequent signs. But also be on the lookout for frequent stomachaches and other gastrointestinal upsets, as these, too, may be allergic responses. (In some instances, bedwetting can be, too.)

Allergy vs. Cold. Allergies are often mistaken for colds when the symptoms involve runny noses and coughs. A sure sign of infection rather than allergy is mucus that is anything but clear. In this instance, echinacea can be called into action (see the section on echinacea earlier in this chapter for guidance on how best to use this immune-stimulating herb).

However, if the symptoms are allergy based, then your child's immune system is already overstimulated, and you would not wish to increase that response with echinacea. This is when soothing, anti-inflammatory properties of herbs help calm the overactive immune system.

The child with a tendency toward food intolerances and environmental sensitivities often exhibits certain characteristics around the eyes, such as puffiness, dark circles, or creases below the eyes.

I prefer to use the terms "sensitivities" or "intolerances" rather than "allergies" to avoid narrowly defining a child's discomfort by the technical biological response usually associated with the word "allergy."

Chemical Sensitivities. Whatever term you use, allergies or sensitivities occur when the body is irritated by a substance. This can be an inhalant, such as dust, mold spores, or pollens, or a chemical like detergent, fabric additives, fragrances, drugs, or food.

If your child's sensitivity is due to a chemical, you'll need to play detective to find the offending substance.

Look in the health food store for a detergent containing the least amount of chemicals. Avoid fabric softeners, commercial bubble baths, deodorant soaps. Use natural, chemical-free soaps for bathing. Avoid products containing fragrance (commonly found in soaps, lotions, and hair products). Some vitamins contain problematic chemicals and dyes.

Food Sensitivities. If your child's sensitivity is due to a food, take heart: this is one of the easiest factors to control. Think not? Well, it's certainly easier than controlling the air they breathe or the thoughts they think! If you eliminate foods that weaken their energy fields, especially during unavoidable exposures (such as peak pollen-producing months), you may find your child can better tolerate the exposure. How do you know which foods weaken their energy fields? Read about food testing in Appendix C and you will be able to pinpoint exactly which foods they are. (Note: whether or not the sensitivity is caused by a food, often the offending food will exacerbate a reaction to another kind of allergen.)

Dairy can be a mucus-forming and mucus-thickening food. If your child exhibits an inability to handle excess mucus, or has breathing difficulties due to nasal or chest congestion, remove milk and cheese from his diet.

For many children, soy milk and soy cheese are good calcium-rich replacements. But always test the soy first as some children do not tolerate it well. Alternatives to soy milk are rice milk and almond milk, both found in health food stores.

Hive-Reducing Tea

A sudden skin reaction, such as hives, is a response to toxic material in the bloodstream. To clear the toxin quickly, and to stop its manifestation in the skin, give your child red clover tea several times a day. This can be had warm or cold, or frozen into ice pops during the summer months. See Chapter 7 for further discussion of hives.

Helpful Botanicals

- ⚘ The nutrients vitamin C and bioflavonoids (substances found in the inner rind of citrus fruits) are helpful in controlling allergic responses. Nettles is a plant high in minerals as well as vitamin C and the bioflavonoids. One way to include nettles in your child's diet is to steam the delicious young spring leaves of the nettles plant and serve it as a vegetable. The freeze-dried form of nettles (available from the herb company Eclectic Institute) can be taken in capsules on a daily basis and is effective in preventing the upper respiratory symptoms associated with hay fever.

- ⚘ When the eyes are irritated due to pollen and mold spores, Dr. Christopher's Herbal Eyebright Formula can bring relief. See Chapter 5 for specific directions on how to use this healing eye treatment.

- ⚘ The expectorant and anti-inflammatory properties of fenugreek seeds can help relieve congestion, reduce postnasal drip, and soothe an irritated throat. If your child is able to safely chew on seeds, give ½–1 teaspoon of pleasant-tasting fenugreek seeds to suck on, chew up, and swallow. If preferred, a warm or cooled tea may be made with the seeds (see Appendix A for how to prepare a decoction). Fenugreek may be given three times a day until symptoms are diminished.

- ⚘ Anise seeds' sweet licorice flavor can be enjoyed in the same manner as fenugreek seeds. Anise soothes the mucus membranes of the upper respiratory tract as well as the digestive tract.

Bee Pollen

German studies have shown that the pollen in honey survives the digestive processes to reach the bloodstream. In a study to determine if pollen solutions could relieve hayfever and allergy-related asthma symptoms in children, 84% responded favorably. The researchers concluded that eating pollen-laden honey could desensitize a child similar to the way allergy injections do.

In his book, *Folk Medicine,* Vermont folk physician, Dr. D. C. Jarvis recommends eating local honey for pollen allergy relief.

- ❀ Locate a beekeeper in your area. Honey derived from local pollens may help to desensitize your child.
- ❀ A teaspoon of honey or honeycomb chewed daily in allergy season and a few times a week for several months prior to allergy season may help to alleviate sensitivity to local pollen and mold spores.

Cell Salts

Ferr. Phos. is always given to support the nervous system. Other cell salts may be appropriate in addition to Ferr. Phos., depending upon your child's symptoms. See Appendix F on cell salts for a suggested repertory.

BEDWETTING

Food Sensitivities

Quite often, bedwetting can be the result of food sensitivities. See Appendix C, Food Testing, to determine which foods your child should avoid.

This issue aside, there are several approaches to take when it comes to bedwetting. First, limit the intake of fluids in the late afternoon and early evening. Also, be sure that your child is voiding completely. If medical examination reveals no physical anomalies that require correction, giving parsley and juniper berry tea daily may help tone and cleanse the kidneys and bladder, helping them to function more efficiently.

Parsley and Juniper Berry Tea

- ❧ Simmer a handful of fresh, flat-leaf parsley and 2 teaspoons fresh or dried juniper berries in 1½ cups water for 15 minutes.
- ❧ Dose according to your child's weight twice a day (see Chapter 3 for dosing guidelines).
- ❧ The tea can be stored in your refrigerator for up to 3 days, and can be served warm or cold.

Remedies to Calm a Nervous Constitution

If you believe that your child's bedwetting stems from nervous agitation:

- ❧ Add a teaspooon of dried chamomile or lemon balm to the parsley and juniper berry tea at the end of the simmering process. Steep for 10 minutes before straining out all the herbs.
- ❧ Consult with a Bach Flower practitioner for a formula personalized to your child (see Appendix I for more on Bach Flower Essences).
- ❧ Consult a homeopathic practitioner for a remedy designed to balance your child's constitution (see Appendix G for locating a homeopath near you).
- ❧ Cell salts may be the magic solution for your child (see Appendix F for further discussion).

Chiropractic

Finally, for some children, chiropractic adjustments of subluxated (misaligned) vertebrae may be the answer to bedwetting.

YEAST/FUNGAL PROBLEMS

Nail Fungus

The simplest, most direct approach to eliminating fingernail or toe-
nail fungus is to use tea tree oil, a highly antifungal, antiseptic essential oil from the Australian tea tree.

- Mix equal parts tea tree oil and a carrier oil such as almond or
  sunflower.
- Apply a couple of drops to the affected area in the morning
  and at bedtime. Keep this up for several weeks or months, if
  necessary.
- If this dilution is too irritating to your child's skin, increase the
  proportion of carrier oil.
- Never give tea tree oil to your child internally, as even a small
  amount can be highly toxic; it is perfectly safe, however, for
  external use.

If the nail does not respond to this one-step approach, then the
addition of internal antifungal herbs is necessary to remove the fungus from the bloodstream.

- Acidophilus (see below).
- Garlic. The adult dose is 2 or 3 cloves a day, 20 drops of garlic
  oil 3 times a day, or 2 tablets of deodorized garlic tablets or garlic perles 3 times a day. See guidelines on dosing in Chapter 3
  to find the amount suitable to your child's weight.
- Black walnut extract (made from the hull and available at health
  food stores). The adult dose is ½ teaspoon in ½ cup warm water,
  twice a day. Dose according to your child's weight. Black walnut
  must be taken for 3 months to completely eliminate the fungus
  from the bloodstream.
- Sugar feeds fungus so be sure to limit its presence in your
  child's diet.

I had a year-long, intimate relationship with black walnut extract. I foolishly gardened without gloves and developed a fungus in one of my fingernails. To compound the problem, I ignored the fungus for too long, and it became so serious that I was actually about to lose the nail. I used black walnut until the symptoms cleared (my nail was inflamed, painful, and itchy), and then stopped only to have the symptoms return. I repeated the therapy until symptoms ceased—only to have them appear in another finger, then later, on the other hand! It took me close to a year to realize that a continuous three-month therapy was required to eliminate the fungus from my body, even though the outward symptoms had quickly disappeared.

Candidiasis

Friendly bacteria and yeast live in ecological balance in the intestinal tract. Antibiotics are challenging to a child's developing immune system. They often kill off the good guys along with the bad and upset this delicate balance. When the good guys—the friendly bacteria that keep the yeast in check—are reduced, the naturally occurring yeast has an opportunity to overgrow, wreaking havoc on your child's immune system.

Candida, a systemic fungal/yeast organism, can be experienced in a variety of ways. Intestinal bloating, fatigue, itchy skin, mood swings, headaches, vaginal infections, urinary tract infections, weight gain, itchy ears, itchy eyes, mouth sores, thrush, and diaper rash are among the most common manifestations. Systemic yeast indicates that the immune system is suffering a challenge.

- ❀ Diluted tea tree oil may be used topically where appropriate.
- ❀ Black walnut and garlic, as described above, are important herbs in ridding the body of candida.
- ❀ I would also recommend adding acidophilus in liquid or tablet form. Acidophilus is the concentrated form of the active culture in yogurt; it repopulates the intestinal tract with friendly bacteria (the "good guys"). It is easily found in health food stores.

Finally, food sensitivities sometimes can be the result of candida. This is because candida can cause irritation in the intestinal tract, making the intestinal wall more permeable to potential food allergens—substances that are toxic to your child's immune system. In full-blown cases of candida, certain foods may need to be avoided. Consult one of the many books on the market for further information on a candida diet for your child.

Supporting Antibiotic Therapy to Prevent Candida

- ❀ Acidophilus should always accompany antibiotic therapy (give to your child 3 times a day, keeping it away from the antibiotic by 1 hour, before or after, taking), and for 3 weeks, 3 times a day following the completion of the antibiotic. Give the last dose of the day right before bedtime so that the good bacteria have a chance to grow unimpeded overnight.
- ❀ Since the antibiotic is stressing the body as it does its job of killing off bacteria, echinacea can accompany the antibiotic therapy and be given 10 days on and 4 days off for a few weeks posttreatment to support the immune system.
- ❀ Be sure your child has plenty of water to drink and is moving the bowels daily. The addition of warm lemonade may be helpful, made with freshly squeezed lemons and a small amount of honey in warm water. Fruits, vegetables, and other fiber-rich foods will help keep the eliminative system moving well.
- ❀ Sugar feeds bacteria, so limit its presence in your child's diet.

Applications

SUPPOSITORIES

In some cases it is more appropriate (and easier) to dose your child with an herb rectally. If you do so, the herb will be absorbed directly into the bloodstream, bypassing the digestive system. This method works especially well if your child is vomiting and cannot take anything by mouth.

How to Make an Herbal Suppository

- ❀ In a shallow dish, mix finely powdered herbs with melted cocoa butter (purchased in a health food store).
- ❀ Refrigerate until hardened.
- ❀ Scoop a teaspoon of the hardened herbs into your hands and roll between your palms to soften into snakelike lengths. Cut into 1" pieces. Lay out on wax paper, refrigerate to reharden.
- ❀ When you are ready to use the suppository, insert it into your child's rectum gently.
- ❀ Hold the buttocks closed for a few minutes to allow the body's heat to disperse the herbs.

HOW TO PREPARE A MEDICINAL TEA

Medicinal teas are prepared differently from the teas we take as everyday beverages. The following guidelines provide the information you need to obtain maximal results from herbal teas.

Infusions/Using Dried Herbs

The more delicate parts of a plant—its leaves, buds, flowers, and stems—are best prepared as a steeped infusion.

- ❀ As a general rule, pour one cup boiled water over one teaspoon herb.
- ❀ Cover, and steep for 15 to 30 minutes, or until cool. Strain before serving.
- ❀ If you are using powdered herbs, use ½ teaspoon to the cup of boiled water.

After many years of trying out various techniques, my favorite way to make an herbal infusion is to use a coffee press.

- ❀ Place the dried herb in the bottom of the glass container, add boiled water.
- ❀ Cover with the press's strainer/plunger top, and steep for the recommended time.
- ❀ Covering the press with a tea cozy will help keep the liquid warm.
- ❀ When it is ready, plunge the top, and the herb will be pressed to the bottom, leaving a clear infusion to drink.

Always be sure to use stainless steel, glass, or enameled cookware and strainers—never aluminum, as this can actually contaminate the herb.

Steam-distilled water (purchased in the supermarket, health food store, or made at home—see Appendix G for resource) is the best medium for an infusion or decoction because it draws more of the plant's medicinal properties into the solution. I have read that as much as 30% more of the plant's chemical constituents are absorbed in the presence of distilled water. If distilled water is not available, bottled or tap water may be used.

Infusions/Using Fresh Herbs

- ✿ Use twice as much fresh herb as dried.
- ✿ Bruise the fresh herb well with a mortar and pestle. This procedure helps break down the plant's capillary walls, releasing the beneficial juices.
- ✿ Decoct the herb using the following directions.

Decoctions/Using Fresh or Dried Herbs

The seeds, bark, and root of a plant need a bit more coaxing to release their healing properties than its aerial parts. For this reason, I recommend a simmering, rather than steeping, process.

- ✿ Simmer 1 tablespoon plant material in 1½ cups water for 15 minutes, keeping pot partially covered.
- ✿ Reduce liquid (by simmering) to 1 cup. Strain and serve.

EQUIVALENCIES

One cup = 8 ounces
One pint = 16 ounces
One quart = 32 ounces
1 teaspoon = ⅛ ounce = 60 drops = 4.5 milliliters

ENCAPSULATED HERBS

When you encapsulate your powdered herbs, use size "00" capsules, available in any health food store. It is very easy to fill a capsule with powdered herbs, as no special equipment is required.

- ✿ Place the powdered material in a small bowl, open a capsule, and fill it by pressing the openings of both ends into the herb.
- ✿ Close the capsule by pushing the ends together.

To help your child learn how to easily swallow a capsule:

- ❀ Coat it with something slippery like a combination of a vegetable or nut oil and/or syrup.
- ❀ Capsules may be opened into applesauce, pudding, or yogurt, or their contents may be mixed into a liquid.

COMPRESSES

A compress is an external, topical therapy used for headaches, tummyaches, menstrual cramps, inflamed skin, or any aching body part.

- ❀ To prepare a compress, soak a clean white cloth or gauze in an herbal tea, or liquid extract or essential oil that has been diluted in water.
- ❀ Press out all excess liquid and apply to the affected area for 20–30 minutes.
- ❀ If the treatment calls for keeping the compress in place overnight, you may wish to cover it with plastic wrap to keep it moist.
- ❀ To keep a compress warm, cover it with a hot water bottle.

POULTICES

Although the name sounds quite ancient, a poultice is simply a compress that uses the whole moistened herb rather than its liquid infusion.

- ❀ To prepare a poultice, place the freshly macerated, or dried herb that has been moistened, between strips of gauze, or apply it directly to the skin.
- ❀ Adding water to powdered herbs transforms them into an easy-to-apply paste.

- Affix the herbal poultice to the skin by binding it with roller gauze or a clean cloth and surgical tape. (I have found that the surgical tape with the best holding power that is also non-irritating to the skin comes in rolls of shiny cloth, and is usually sold in surgical pharmacies without a dispenser.)
- Plastic wrap may be used to keep it moist overnight.
- For a problem that requires more than one treatment, make a fresh poultice with each application for maximum effect.

Castor Oil Pack

- Fold a piece of white, wool flannel (some health food stores have this item, or see Appendix G for resources) to comfortably cover the affected area and put enough cold-pressed castor oil on it so it is moistened, but not runny.
- Apply to affected area and cover with a hot water bottle.
- To keep it in place, first spread a bath towel on the bed, place your child on top of it, and wrap it around both the child and the flannel cloth and hot water bottle.
- Leave the pack on for an hour, repeating application every couple of hours, until your child feels better.
- When you are finished using the castor oil pack, the residual oil should be cleaned from the skin using a wash of ½ teaspoon baking soda dissolved in ½ cup water. This is to prevent the skin from reabsorbing any toxins the castor oil may have pulled to its surface.
- The flannel may be stored in a glass jar. Do not wash it. The next time you need it, simply add more castor oil.

INHALATIONS

Upper respiratory congestion may be relieved by inhaling herbal steams.

- Place a heated tea or 4 drops essential oil diluted in hot water in a shallow pan.

- Form a tent with a terrycloth towel and have your child sit close and inhale deeply.
- The addition of several drops of an essential oil to a vaporizer can infuse your child's room with antimicrobial properties.

HOW TO STORE AND PRESERVE HERBAL REMEDIES

The best place to store any herbal medicine is in a dry, cool closet like the one you use for linens. The worst place is the steamy bathroom medicine cabinet, or near a hot stove or oven.

Liquid Extracts

When stored in a dark, cool closet, liquid extracts can have a shelf life of several years. Refrigeration is not required.

Dried Herbs and Capsules

Stored in tightly capped, dark glass or opaque plastic bottles away from heat and moisture, herbs will retain their freshness for as long as two years.

Herbal Teas

After you have made an herb into an infusion or decoction, you can store it covered, in the refrigerator, for up to three days.

Where to Get Your Herbs

If you choose to grow your own:

- You may begin with seeds, seedlings, or young plants purchased at a commercial greenhouse.
- Be certain you are growing the exact variety you desire for specific healing purposes by checking the Latin name first. Sage,

for instance, comes in many varieties, but only *Salvia offici-nalis* will do for its astringent and diaphoretic properties.

❧ Do not apply chemicals to your lawn or garden when you choose to grow herbs as medicinals. (Naturally, the same warning applies when receiving gifts from someone else's garden. Double-check the Latin name and make sure that the plant has not been treated with chemicals.)

If you pick your own herbs:

❧ You must always use a botanical guide. Otherwise, you might pick something poisonous or take the wrong herb altogether, thus depriving your child of the intended plant's valuable therapeutic effect.

❧ An excellent book to consult is *A Field Guide to Medicinal Plants: Eastern and Central North America* by James A. Duke and Steven Foster (Houghton Mifflin, 1992). This book provides wonderful, easy-to-identify pictures and comments that help you select the herb you want.

❧ Extremely important note: You must be certain that the area in which you are foraging for herbs has not been chemically treated in any way, for the reasons I mention above. There is a saying among mushroom hunters that applies well here. There are old mushroom hunters, and there are bold mushroom hunters, but there are no old, bold mushroom hunters. Herb harvester, beware!

If you are purchasing herbs:

❧ Dried herbs, herbal products, and formulations may be purchased from your local herbalist or health food store as long as the merchant is willing to guarantee that they are (where possible) nonirradiated.

❧ The dried herbs and spices you can buy on your supermarket's shelves have, in all probability, been subject to radiation. Irradiation, a topic of great dispute as it relates to our food supply, has been permitted for herbs and spices for many years. The herb's vibration and life force are altered when the plant is irradiated, rendering its medicinal properties unpredictable and questionable. Although we view plants as physical substances, there is an unseen (though measurable) vibrational/energetic quality to them that contributes to their healing profiles. For this reason, I recommend that you save the supermarket herbs for cooking. A pinch of irradiated herb for use in the kitchen will do no harm, while a handful of irradiated herbs for healing might.

Characteristics of Herbs

It is the chemical composition of herbs that makes them effective. Their therapeutic action can be grouped into the following categories:

Adaptogens

See "tonics."

Alteratives

Herbs that purify the bloodstream and, in turn, cleanse organs. These detoxifying herbs include red clover, echinacea, barberry, and yarrow.

Anthelmintics

See "vermifuges."

Astringents

Herbs that condense and firm tissue as required with hemorrhoids. Astringent herbs cleanse mucus from tissue and help to dry up fluids, as in diarrhea. Examples: mullein, cayenne, and white oak bark.

Carminatives

Herbs that help eliminate intestinal gas. A colicky baby would be given fennel, dill, or anise.

Cathartics

Herbs that cleanse waste matter from the intestinal tract and stimulate peristaltic action helping the bowels function more effectively. Senna is an example of an extremely cathartic herb, while turkey rhubarb is a very mild one.

Cholagogues

Herbs that cleanse the gallbladder. Examples include barberry, dandelion, and goldenseal.

Demulcents

Herbs that soothe due to their mucilaginous composition. Examples: comfrey, aloe, and calendula.

Diaphoretics

Herbs that are taken hot to stimulate perspiration and, thereby, the release of toxins, as is desired in colds and flu. When taken cold, diaphoretic herbs help diminish the flow of fluids. A nursing mother, when ready to wean her child, could use a cold sage tea to stop the flow of fluids.

Diuretics

Herbs that cleanse the kidneys and bladder by stimulating the flow of urine. One urinates more frequently or more fully when taking diuretic herbs. Examples: juniper berry, parsley, uva ursi.

Emmenagogues

Herbs that balance the menstrual flow. Examples include blessed thistle, wild yam root, and chaste berry.

Expectorants

Herbs that help the mucus membranes of the chest area cleanse and release excess phlegm, which accompanies bronchitis and pneumonia. Examples include mullein, garlic, and cayenne.

Nervines

Herbs to help relax the muscles and nourish the nervous system — actions that make nervines helpful for sleep problems. Examples: valerian root, hops, and passionflower.

Stimulants

Herbs that promote circulation, thereby increasing energy. A peppermint bath would be ideal to start the day but too stimulating for bedtime. Examples are cayenne, ginger, and peppermint.

Tonics

Herbs that gently strengthen and tone the organs. A uterine tonic would, for instance, be given to a female having menstrual irregularities; a digestive tonic in the case of poor assimilation of nutrients; and a cardiac tonic for someone with heart problems. Tonics can be used safely long-term.

Vermifuges

Herbs to help cleanse the body of parasites. Examples: garlic, black walnut, wormwood.

Food Testing

There are several ways to determine if your child has a food sensitivity. The most popular method is the elimination diet. In this method, all suspect foods are eliminated from the child's diet until symptoms disappear. This may take up to a week or two. Then one food is reintroduced for 3 days while a detailed journal of the child's physical responses is kept. This continues until all foods have been tested. Often, combinations of foods also have to be tested because the body may be able to tolerate them individually but not together.

As you can readily see, this can be a long, drawn-out affair, often complicated by the interference of variables such as exposure to animal dander or pollens, illness, or mood swings, any of which can alter the body's response to a particular food.

The method I've used for many years, both with clients and my own children, is known by several names—kinesiology, muscle testing, and energy testing. The principle is to remove from the diet whatever weakens the body's electrical system. The strength of the electrical system is measured by a muscle response to the food in question. It's a very simple procedure to learn and put into action. It is, I believe, the most reliable method for testing food sensitivities. Also, rather than relying upon our intellect, in muscle testing we allow the child's body to communicate its own strengths and weaknesses. No matter how well educated I am in this area, I much prefer to let the body's intelligence dictate a plan of action.

How to Test Foods

- ✿ The easiest testing circuits are the wrist/thigh position or thumb/pinky connection (description to follow).
- ✿ For infants, or children too young to reliably hold a position, surrogate testing (description to follow) works equally well.
- ✿ Whichever technique you use, always get a baseline reading first by testing without the food present and then again with your child holding the food.
- ✿ If a food tests well, you are looking for the muscle connection to stay as strong as it was in the baseline test, without the food.
- ✿ If holding the food weakens the connection, the food is not having a strengthening effect upon the body and should be eliminated from the diet.
- ✿ Later, as a result of healing herbs and elimination of challenging substances in the external and internal environments, the child's body will become stronger and less reactive. This is when you can try reintroducing previously eliminated foods.
- ✿ You may find they can be tolerated when not eaten in combination with other offending foods. For example, a child with wheat and dairy sensitivities may now be able to have a bowl of macaroni without cheese.

There are many things in life that can weaken the body over which we have limited or no control; these include environmental pollution and emotional stress. It is especially important, then, that the daily nourishment of food and liquid helps create a balanced internal environment, thereby rendering the body less reactive to those things we cannot control. Muscle-testing your child's food-and-drink intake can help you create the best program to support that balance. Since the knowledge derived from the testing is immediately accessed, you can always be assured of giving your child the foods that are strengthening his or her body by periodically retesting them. I consider muscle testing a tool to help achieve peace of mind—both for the parent and the child!

Wrist/Thigh Position

- ✿ Stand to the left of your child, both of you facing forward.
- ✿ Both of you space your feet just wide enough to comfortably keep yourselves erect when gently pulled.
- ✿ Have your child place the left wrist against the left thigh, with elbow slightly bent.
- ✿ Slip the index and middle fingers of your right hand behind the child's wrist. (If necessary, your positions may be reversed, with you to the right of your child.) (See figure #8.)
- ✿ Ask your child to firmly press the wrist against the thigh.
- ✿ Gently at first, pull against the wrist as your child resists your pull.
- ✿ Increase the strength of your pull until the child's wrist finally weakens. This gives you a baseline test, indicating the strength of your child's natural resistance, against which you will compare future tests.
- ✿ When beginning a new session of food testing, always take a baseline reading before testing the food. A person's level of resistance can vary from day to day or even throughout the day, depending upon activities, external influences, etc.
- ✿ Now, have the child hold the food to be tested in the other hand.
- ✿ The energy field of a food can emanate through plastic or

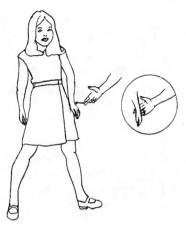

glass, but not through metal. Do not use foods in cans or food that has been wrapped in aluminum foil.

❀ Test the food by pulling on your child's wrist as before. If the wrist easily resists your pull, the food strengthens your child's electrical field.

❀ If your child's strength is obviously weakened when you pull on it, the food's energy field is responsible for the weakened response and should be eliminated from the child's diet for the time being.

When a food first weakens the subject, it can be most surprising. Your child will usually say, "Do it again—I wasn't ready!" To prepare your child for the wrist pull, you can say something like, "hold tight" or "'try to resist my pull." You can make muscle testing a fun activity and even do it in the supermarket. This way, you can avoid buying a food that does not test well.

Thumb/Pinky Connection

❀ Have your child hold the left hand, fingers open, with the palm facing upwards.

❀ Help her connect the left thumb and pinky fingers by putting one nail under the other, creating a circle.

❀ Take a baseline test by putting your two index fingers under

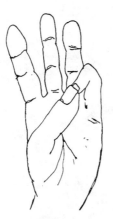

the pads of the thumb/pinky connection, gently trying to separate them. (See figure #9.)

- ❀ Be sure to prepare the child to "hold tight and resist." Remember, this is not a test of your brute strength versus your child's! It is, rather, an energetic test.
- ❀ Proceed by having your child hold the food in the other hand as you test the thumb/pinky connection. The connection will be weakened or strenghtened as described for the wrist/thigh position.

Surrogate Testing

This is the preferred method for testing infants and toddlers for food intolerances.

- ❀ Have another adult wrap their right arm around the baby, holding the food against the baby's body, while you test the adult's thumb/pinky connection. (See figure #10.)
- ❀ It will seem as though you are testing the adult's energy field rather than the baby's, but while the adult is holding the infant, they are actually reflecting the baby's energy field.
- ❀ Always remember to take a baseline reading before testing the food.

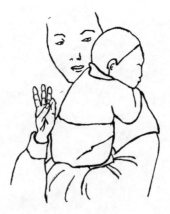

A mother brought her newborn to my office because she was unable to breastfeed, and the child was doing very poorly on prepared formula. I had her bring in every product she could find on the supermarket shelves so that we could see if there was some brand of formula that would agree with the child without putting the infant through the process of ingesting and regurgitating the product (which is what was happening with all formulas the mother had previously tried). Using surrogate testing, we were able to quickly determine that only one of 17 products commercially available strengthened the baby's energy field; this was the one that, in the long run, helped her to thrive.

- ❦ In all testing situations, be conscious of keeping the pressure of your pull at a consistent level of force and resistance.
- ❦ Also, so that your subconscious mind does not affect the outcome, detach yourself emotionally from the food. It should not matter to you that a particular food tests well or not; instead, focus on ascertaining your child's body's response, be it weak or strong. If you feel that you can't detach yourself from the results—many of us do have strong positive and negative associations to foods—then have someone else do the testing for you.

Many health practitioners, including chiropractors and holistic medical doctors, use muscle testing as a diagnostic tool. Although you may find it strange to work with at first, keep practicing until you are comfortable with this most valuable tool. The result will be a wonderful, fun, and easy method for nourishing your child with foods tailored to his or her special needs.

Understanding Toxicity and How It Affects Your Child

Where Do Toxins Come From? We parents tend to view our newborns as the purest reflection of God's/nature's/man's/woman's making. However, these sweet creatures can acquire toxins from their birth mothers while inside the womb. Once they enter our world, babies are exposed to all sorts of foreign invaders, or toxins, and we hope that their little immune systems are prepared to maintain the highest order of protection.

What are some toxins that can invade our children's bodies? As children grow, they are exposed to more and more challenging substances. Contributing factors to toxic overload may include consumption of incompatible foods, ingesting or inhaling drugs, lack of exercise, breathing poor quality air, chronic constipation, drinking impure water, immunizations, undetected residues of viruses, bacteria, fungus, and parasites.

Ironically, what we think of as home improvements or decorating may actually expose your youngster to a plethora of chemicals outgassing from carpeting, paint, wallpaper, and/or furniture. Substances used to keep our homes clean may, in fact, challenge your child's maturing immune system.

Ongoing emotional upset can produce more toxic residue from stress hormones than the body may be equipped to handle. Allergies are a response to substances being treated as unfriendly by the body; these include pollens, animal dander, chemicals, and food by-products.

Ridding the Body of Toxic Waste. How does the body rid itself of toxins? Through its house-cleaning organs. The kidneys and bladder, through urination, remove toxins from active circulation in the bloodstream. It is thus wise to encourage your child to respond to the bladder's call rather than trying to hold it in too long. Drinking lots of good quality water helps the kidneys and bladder flush out toxins more effectively.

One of the liver's myriad functions is to filter toxins. Largely composed of fat cells (which, unfortunately, store toxins all too well), an overburdened liver will eventually perform its filtering processes less efficiently, thereby producing irritation somewhere in the body.

The colon is beautifully designed to rid the body of toxic material. Feeding your child high-fiber foods and lots of good water helps the colon move toxins out of the body. Encourage good bowel habits so that your child has easy eliminations every day. Diarrhea is a first line defense in protecting the body from highly toxic waste.

Our skin releases toxins through perspiration. Exercise helps produce a cleansing perspiration. When your child is feverish, encourage sweating with appropriate herbal teas as a means of releasing toxins.

Cold and flu symptoms should not be pharmaceutically suppressed. They are often another attempt by the body to release toxins. Medicinal herbs, in helping the body to heal itself, will assist in clearing up symptoms.

Toxic Interference. How do toxins interfere with a child's well-being? When your child's body is bogged down with residue, it has difficulty assimilating the nutrition it receives and healthfully carrying on with its daily functions. Although many variables are responsible for protecting the body from scavenging microorganisms like viruses and parasites, they are more easily accepted into a body that has already been compromised by the presence of toxins.

Chronic constipation may continue to circulate toxins in the blood, producing flulike symptoms; exit them through the skin, developing into acne, cysts, or boils; cause chronic irritation in the bladder; or inflame mucus membranes, resulting in chronic respiratory infections. Ongoing fatigue and depression may also be the results of toxic wastes affecting the brain and central nervous system.

Antibiotics: A Mixed Blessing. In the presence of severe bacterial infection, antibiotics can be lifesavers. They are not, however, effective, nor were they designed for the treatment of viruses. In a *New York Times* (August 3, 1999) interview with Dr. Paul A. Offit, Chief of Infectious Diseases at Children's Hospital of Philadelphia, and Dr. Bonnie Fass-Offitt, a pediatrician in private practice, about the overuse of antibiotics, they indicated that in 100 children with fever, about 90% will be due to viruses rather than bacteria. Of these 100 children, 60–70% will receive antibiotics even though they will do nothing to relieve the symptoms or hasten recovery from the viral infection.

The use of an antibiotic to prevent secondary bacterial infection is a commonly used protocol in the presence of viral infection. This is important for the child prone to developing fluid congestion in the areas of the chest or ears with a tendency to settle there and become bacterially infected.

However, according to the doctors interviewed in the *New York Times*. article, parental pressure upon the child's doctor is often cited as the cause for the inappropriately prescribed antibiotics.

When you do not know how to help relieve your child's symptoms, panic can set in, promoting unwise responses and choices.

If parents are versed in the use of natural remedies, they may be able to responsibly take charge of the medically diagnosed viral infection before it gets in charge of the child's body.

Overuse of antibiotics may cause other toxic situations to develop. The liver can overload in an attempt to process the toxic residue of repeated antibiotic therapy. The ecology of the colon becomes disturbed by having its army of friendly bacteria reduced. This allows naturally occurring yeast to overgrow, and a multitude of disturbances in the body can result.

Rebuilding Health

There is good news here. Upon completion of antibiotic therapy, the toxic residue can be processed out of the body by eating healthy foods and giving your child herbs that help cleanse the organs.

- ✿ You can help your child rebuild health by planning a wellness-promoting diet. Eating vegetables, fruits, grains, nuts, and seeds—with the addition, if you prefer, of small amounts of animal protein such as fish and chicken—helps the body to more easily perform its digestive processes.
- ✿ "Junk foods" and large amounts of the more difficult-to-digest proteins such as red meat and dairy make it harder for the body to efficiently carry on with its digestive functions.
- ✿ Cleansing with herbs, drinking lots of good quality water, and plenty of exercise all greatly enhance the body's well-being.
- ✿ Helping your child better handle emotional stress via meditation and positive thinking can bring untold benefits now and for their future lives.

And one more thing . . . please reread this chapter and see how it might apply to your own lifestyle. The easiest way to grow healthy children is to be a reflection of what you want for them and the behaviors you seek them to adopt.

Internal Cleansing

We make sure our children's bodies get washed, but how about their inner bodies? As a rule, it's a good holistic health practice to cleanse your bloodstream and liver with the change of seasons. Our bodies are hard at work doing their best, day in and day out. How about giving them a helping hand?

If your child tends to get a lot of colds, has body odor, smelly feet, bad breath, or many skin problems, all for no apparent health or psychological reason, it may well be time to pay a little attention to the liver.

The liver is the organ that (in addition to its many other responsibilities) filters the toxins of the body. If it has been overloaded with
toxic residue from foods, stress, medication, and/or the environment, the liver may do its job a little less efficiently—circulating toxins through the bloodstream and into other organs. This is when
trouble starts brewing.

Remember "Andrea's Rule of Three"? (See page 3.) Three weeks
is the proper time for cleansing. During this period, you should
focus on healthy eating, eliminating junk food, and giving your
child's body a rest from unnecessary toxic residues. This is the
time to give her lots of good water to drink, preferably filtered or
distilled.

Herbal Cleansers

- Yarrow tea gently cleanses the liver. Give your child 1 or 2
  cups a day. Yarrow can taste rather bitter, but sweetens up
  nicely with the addition of just a touch of honey.
- Beets are excellent blood cleansers. Serve ½ a beet a day juiced
  (with other juices, like carrot or apple), grated into salad, or
  lightly steamed. Beets are also delicious when mixed with
  mashed avocado, and the resultant color is striking too!
- Cinnamon is very good for the liver. Find delicious foods that
  can benefit from the addition of cinnamon. Among my family's favorites are cinnamon toast, rice pudding, sweet potatoes,
  oatmeal, and applesauce.
- Watermelon cleanses the liver, kidneys, colon, and bladder.
  Choose a hot summer day and call it "Watermelon Day"—eating nothing but watermelon all day long. It's a great cleansing
  fast for the whole family, and you can have seed spitting con-
  tests to make the whole experience more fun.
- Organic grapes are good blood cleansers. The fall Concord
  grapes with seeds are the ones to eat, though grapes with seeds
  aren't especially pleasant for the younger child.
- Red clover tea makes a nice, gentle blood cleanser. Give it to
  your child up to 3 times a day in ½- to 1-cup servings. This works

well either warm, or cold, as an iced herbal tea. Better yet, freeze
the tea into ice pops for a really healthy snack or dessert!
* Fall burdock root and spring dandelion leaves are nice liver-
cleansing additions at the appropriate times of the year.
* For a detailed program of detoxifying herbs, see pages
167–169.

APPENDIX E

Healing Imagery

Healing imagery has played an important role in medicine throughout many parts of the world for centuries. With the advent of modern medical thinking, its popular acceptance as a healing tool in the United States began to wane, along with herbal medicine. However, both modalities have remained alive in Europe and much of the rest of the world, and are enjoying a resurgence in America.

The growing field of psychoneuroimmunology posits that the mind and body are one entity, the bodymind. The mind's influence upon the body can be harnessed for the purpose of healing by creating images of wellness. Medical studies have in fact revealed that people tend to heal faster and more fully when they take an active part in their own treatment.

Basketball teams have used creative imagery during practices. In a controlled study, one half of a team engaged in their regular 30-minute daily practice of foul-line shooting. The other half of the team *imagined* the practicing of foul shots for 30 minutes a day. Impressively, the imaging players scored more foul shots during their games! Divers, figure skaters, and Olympic athletes have used imaging quite successfully.

The mind can experience an event just as real as if the body were actually going through it. An imagined situation can be as concrete an event as one experienced directly by the senses of the physical body. In a situation perceived as potentially threatening, the heart will beat faster as if it were engaged in the actual experience. Adjust the mind's imagery about the perceived threat, and the body will respond accordingly.

234

Here's how visual imagery can be used to better our health:

✿ The immune system can be visualized destroying disease-producing cells.

✿ Patients are asked to see the immune system as an army of white knights who attack invaders; or they may think of them as computerized "pac men," eating up the bad guys.

✿ Cysts and tumors can be creatively imagined to be shrinking until they have vanished completely. A tumor could be seen as a ball of light reducing in size until it has disappeared.

✿ Projected fears can be reimagined with happy, productive outcomes.

✿ The healing of wounds can be accelerated by enhancing cellular communication with imagery. The wound might be envisioned in a sickly gray color, turning healthy pink as it heals.

✿ Headaches can be calmed by visualizing soothing blue light bathing the head.

Gerald Epstein, M.D., author of *Healing Visualizations: Creating Healing Through Imagery* (Bantam, 1989) and *Healing Into Immortality* (Bantam, 1994 and Acmi, 1996) tells of a visualization he gave to a patient with eczema. He had the man imagine his fingers becoming palm leaves that he placed on his face. He was told to "feel the flow of water and milk becoming a river of honey that heals the area." The man was further instructed to "leave a drop of oil on the healed area after finishing," seeing his face totally cleared in his mind's eye. He did this exercise three times a day for 21 days at approximately the same time each day. The man's face improved considerably, and he used a similar approach for other parts of his body.

Of course, the benefit of working with someone like Dr. Epstein, who is a psychiatrist, is that his professional training lends itself to exploring underlying causes of illness, and allows him to create specific visualizations to deal with the medical problem at hand.

You can help your child develop just the right healing imagery for his or her particular situation by talking about the problem in an imaginary context. As you will see in the following example, children are far more creative than we are—also, their minds are freer in many ways—and will develop just the right visualization for their needs.

Eight-year-old Matthew suffered from daily headaches. Food, emotions, and environment were all taken into consideration; still, his headaches persisted. I asked Matthew to tell me what color his headaches were, how big or little his head felt when he had them, what color he felt would calm them down. We also discussed whether or not there was a sound or taste associated with them. At the end of our discussion Matthew determined that his healing imagery was seeing himself lying by a stream of blue water, where an angel was continuously pouring healing water over his head. A blue cloud of angels played pretty music as his head was soothed and free of discomfort.

Before beginning an imagery exercise, teach your child how to breathe out, then in, slowly and rhythmically, with eyes closed. Matthew was instructed to begin each visualization with slow, rhythmic breathing—breathing out, then in, 3 times. As he breathed deeply, he mentally stated his intention to be rid of his headache. The actual imagery was meant to take place quickly: He took a breath and lay down in the water . . . took a breath and saw the angel bathing his hair . . . took a breath, saw and heard the cloud of angels . . . took a breath and felt his head cleared. He took three breaths in this healed state and ended the imagery by opening his eyes.

Matthew first discovered that he could stop the headaches with his imagery and later found that he could prevent them as well. By our next visit, his daily headaches were history.

Healing visualizations can be an excellent adjunct to other forms of therapy. They are wonderful ways to engage your children, empowering them in their own path to wellness.

In his book, Dr. Epstein describes the components of a healing visualization: intention, quieting, cleansing, changing. An adaptation of this profile would look like this:

1. Quieting
   ⚜ Create a peaceful, quiet atmosphere.
   ⚜ Take the phone off the hook.

❀ Have your child sit or lie down.
❀ Breathe slowly and rhythmically with your child.
❀ When this feels comfortable, have your child breathe out, then in, 3 times.

2. Intention
   ❀ Have your child state an intention for healing, acknowledging that this is his choice.
   ❀ Help him to understand that by giving his inner body a direction, he is cleansing it to function more healthfully through the power of his mind.

3. Cleansing
   ❀ Discuss your child's discomfort in terms of color, sound, taste, smell, as well as its size, shape, and how it feels.
   ❀ What color, sound, etc. would make it disappear?
   ❀ Does an active participant need to be called in (like a white knight or pac man or angel)?
   ❀ Allow your child to be totally involved in creating his or her own healing imagery.

4. Changing
   ❀ Encourage your child to describe the area in its healthy state.
   ❀ This may be represented by a new color, shape, sound, or other image.

5. Frequency
   ❀ Depending upon the situation, the imagery may be repeated every few hours, or just once or twice a day, for an ongoing period of time; as needed.
   ❀ Caution! Repeating the imagery too often is like telling the body "this isn't working."
   ❀ It is important to tell the body how you want it to be and then let go so it can do its own healing work.

Cell Salts

I have used cell salts with my own children to treat nasal congestion and colds. They are an excellent adjunct to herbal therapy. The cell salts help stop the irritation of runny nose, ease congestion, and relieve headaches; as such, they nicely complement echinacea (to build the immune system) and garlic (an antimicrobial). Cell salts are easy to travel with and pleasant to take.

According to biochemical theory, cells are composed of water, organic, and inorganic substances. The water and organic substances are used by the inorganic substances, known as cell or tissue salts, to promote cellular function. Generally, our bodies spontaneously compensate when there is a deficiency of any kind. When this does not occur (typically when the body is under some sort of emotional or psychological stress) symptoms can arise in the presence of a cell-salt deficiency. Thus, it is the nature of the symptom, rather than its medical name, that determines which cell salt is required to return equilibrium to our bodies.

To determine the cell salt you need to use, you must consult a repertory of symptoms and substances. The small size of *The Biochemic Handbook* (Chapman & Perry, rev. 1994) makes it an easy reference guide, and one that travels well. A more complete compendium may be found in *The Twelve Tissue Remedies of Schuessler* by Boericke and Dewey (B. Jain Publishers (P) Ltd., New Delhi, India, reprinted 1993). Or you can obtain other guides from Homeopathic Educational Services, 2124 Kittredge Street, Berkeley, CA 94704 (800-359-9051).

You can buy cell salts individually or in easy-to-use kits in most health food stores. They are quite inexpensive and very safe to use. I recommend buying a kit that contains small vials of the 12 cell salts.

Dosing Cell Salts

Cell salts are easy to give to any child as they are tiny, sweet-tasting pellets that quickly dissolve in the mouth. Also known as tissue salts, they are purchased in 6X potency at most health food stores.

   ❁ For an infant, dissolve a pellet in a small amount of water, take it up in a dropper, and insert it into the baby's mouth directly under the tongue.

Infants to 2 years	1 pellet
Ages 2–6 years	2 pellets
Ages 6–12 years	3 pellets
Ages 12 and over	4 pellets

Note: Dose 15 minutes before or after food or drink, or the remedy will be antidoted by whatever your child ingests. Cell salts are delicate homeopathic remedies with their own individual vibrations. The vibration of something else ingested could interfere with the activity of the cell salt.

   ❁ In acute situations, dose every 15 minutes, then every 30–60 minutes until your child feels better, then every 3 hours until well.

   ❁ In ongoing, chronic situations, give 3–4 times a day.

   ❁ Cell salts are fragile and should not be handled. To remove the dose, tap into the vial's cap and pour directly into the child's mouth, preferably under the tongue. If a pellet drops, discard it; do not return it to the vial.

Please do not be intimidated by this simple homeopathic family of remedies. It is easy to determine which cell salt is needed, nothing could be easier to administer, and cell salts are much less expensive than over-the-counter cold remedies.

Resource Guide

PRODUCT RESOURCES

❀ Alpine Air of America
220 Reservoir Street
Needham Heights, MA 02194
800–628–2209
(Air purifier/ionizer)

❀ A.R.E.
Association for Research and Enlightenment
P.O. Box 595, Atlantic Avenue
Virginia Beach, VA 23451
804–438–3588
(Resource for Edgar Cayce products)

❀ Boiron-Borneman, Inc
800-BLU-TUBE
(Homeopathic remedies)

❀ Colon 8
IonLabs, Inc.
6545 44th St. N
Pinellas Park, FL 34665
813–527–1072
(Colon cleanser used with herbal detoxification program)

❀ Dr. Christopher's Original Formulas
1195 Spring Creek Place

Springville, UT 84663
800–453–1406
(A good resource for ordering small quantities of dried herbs as
well as Dr. Christopher's products)

❀ Face Rejuvenation
97 Bouton Road
So. Salem, NY 10590
914–763–8889
(For aloe/acne treatment: Aloe whipped with glycerin)

❀ Frontier Natural Products Co-Op
3021 78th Street
P.O. Box 299
Norway, IA 52318
800–669–3275
(Bulk herbs and for ½ oz. and 1 oz. dropper bottles)

❀ Gemma
P.O. Box 68
Trumbull, CT 06611
203–268–2394
(For facial scrub)

❀ Gilberties Herb and Garden Center
7 Sylvan Lane
Westport, CT 06880
203–227–4175
(Fresh herb plants and seeds shipped throughout the country)

❀ Hanna's Herb Shop
805 Walnut Street
Boulder, CO 80302
800–206–6722
(Makes available individual homeopathic remedies for specific
residues as well as herbal teas, extracts, and capsules)

✿ Heritage Products
800–726–2232
(Resource for Edgar Cayce products)

✿ Nature's Therapy Herb Pac
Street Smart Enterprise
P.O. Box 51
Hallwood, VA 223359
757–824–0076
(Hot/cold herbal pack)

✿ Quantum Herbal Products, Ltd.
20 DeWitt Drive
Saugerties, NY 12477
800–348–0398
(Excellent resource for vibrationally enhanced liquid extracts)

✿ Traditional Medicinals
4515 Rose Road
Sebastopol, CA 95472
707–623–8911
(A medicinal tea company offering a wide variety of excellent
formulas, widely found in health food stores)

✿ Waterwise
P.O. Box 494000
Leesburg, FL 34749
352–787–5008
(Water distillers, portable or installed)

RESOURCES FOR LOCATING NATURAL HEALTH PRACTITIONERS

MASTER HERBALIST

A master herbalist is usually well known to the local health food store. Ask the proprietor or a holistic educational center for a recommendation.

NATUROPATHIC PHYSICIAN

A naturopathic physician is one who incorporates natural healing modalities into his/her medical practice. At present, they are only licensed in 11 states: Alaska, Arizona, Connecticut, Hawaii, Maine, Montana, New Hampshire, Oregon, Utah, Vermont, and Washington. When choosing a naturopathic physician, be sure the doctor's degree is from an accredited college or university. Also, please know that some naturopaths do specialize in pediatrics.

For help in locating a naturopathic physician, you can contact their professional organization at 206–298–0125, or sign on to their web site at www.naturopathic.org for a listing by location.

PRACTITIONER SPECIALIZING IN NATURAL REMEDIES FOR LYME DISEASE

Healers Who Share
9068C Marshal Court
Westminster, CO
303-428-4584

HOMEOPATHIC PRACTITIONER

National Center for Homeopathy
801 North Fairfax Street
Alexandria, VA 22314
703-548-7790

Compendium of holistic healthcare practitioners in
NY/NJ/CT

The Holistic Resource Network Directory
P.O. Box 171
South Salem, NY 10590
www.holistic-resource.com

To Find Out More About Medicinal Herbs

The Herb Research Foundation
A nonprofit research/education center
For membership and quarterly newsletter and herb hotline:
1007 Pearl Street, Suite 200
Boulder, CO 80302
303–449–2265

The American Botanical Council
Publishers of *Herbalgram* (a scientific review of botanicals)
P.O. Box 201660
Austin, TX 78720
512–331–8868

The American Holistic Medical Association
4101 Lake Boone Trail, Suite 201
Raleigh, NC 27607
919–787–5181

The American Association of Naturopathic Physicians (AANP)
601 Valley St., Suite 105
Seattle, WA 98102
206–298–0126

Annual Medicinal Herb Symposia:

Gaia Herbs
12 Lancaster County Road
Harvard, MA 01451

Frontier Natural Products Co-Op
P.O. Box 299
Norway, IA 52318
800–669–3275

The American Herbalists Guild
e-mail: ahgoffice@earthlink.net

APPENDIX H

Product Ingredients

Given my training and long-term use of his products with children, I often find myself recommending one of Dr. Christopher's formulas. I keep my work clear of any financial arrangements with natural products companies so that I am free to recommend what I think is best rather than what I am financially connected to. I think this is important so that people feel comfortable with my recommendations.

Dr. Christopher generously shared his formulas with the public, and I wish to carry on that intent. Following is a list of ingredients for each product discussed in this book. They can be ordered from the number given in Appendix G or, if you wish, you can find other similarly formulated products in the health food store. Keep in mind, however, that while other products may have similar ingredients, we don't always know in what quantity they are included.

If you would like to find out about other formulas published by Dr. Christopher, two of his many books are *Childhood Diseases* (Christopher Publications, 1976) and *School of Natural Healing*. You can contact the Christopher organization (see Appendix G) for a complete listing.

Sometimes it is not wise to give a large quantity of an herb but that very same herb may be perfectly safe when given in smaller amounts and balanced in a formula of other herbs. An example of this is comfrey. Comfrey contains alkaloids which can be harmful to the liver when had in large quantity. However, when comfrey is given in small amounts and in formula with other herbs, as it is, for example, in the BF&C formula, it is very safe and a wonderful healing herb. Nature just didn't design comfrey to be had as your main meal!

Many of the following formulas are available in liquid as well as capsule form.

Fen LB *(lower-bowel formula)*

Barberry Bark
Cascara Sagrada Bark
Cayenne Fruit
Ginger Root
Lobelia Herb

Red Raspberry Leaf
Turkey Rhubarb Root
Fennel Seed
Goldenseal Root

Juni-Pars *(kidney-bladder formula)*

Juniper Berries
Parsley Root
Uva Ursi Leaf
Marshmallow Root

Lobelia Herb
Ginger Root
Goldenseal Root

SHA *(sinus, hayfever, allergy formula) (also known as Sinutean)*

Brigham Tea
Marshmallow Root
Goldenseal Root
Chaparral Leaf

Burdock Root
Parsley Root
Lobelia Herb
Cayenne Fruit

Relax-Eze *(nervine formula)*

Black Cohosh Root
Capsicum Fruit
Hops Flowers
Lobelia Herb

Skullcap Herb
Valerian Root
Wood Betony
Mistletoe Herb

Resp-Free *(lung/bronchial formula) (also known as Respratean)*

Comfrey Leaf
Mullein Leaf
Chickweed Herb

Marshmallow Root
Lobelia Herb

Herbal Eyebright Formula *(eye-cleansing formula)*

Bayberry Bark   Red Raspberry Leaf
Eyebright Herb   Cayenne Fruit
Goldenseal Root

Nu Fem *(female reproductive organ formula)*

Goldenseal Root   Ginger Root
Blessed Thistle Herb   Red Raspberry Leaf
Cayenne Fruit   Squawvine Herb
Cramp Bark   Uva Ursi Leaf
False Unicorn Root

BF&C *(bone, flesh & cartilage formula)*

White Oak Bark   Skullcap Herb
Marshmallow Root   Comfrey Leaf
Mullein Leaf   Black Walnut Leaf
Wormwood Herb   Gravel Root
Lobelia Herb

Comfrey-Mullein-Garlic Syrup *(cough formula)*

Comfrey Root   Garlic Syrup
Mullein Leaf   Vegetable Glycerine

CMM Ointment *(skin formula)*

Comfrey Root   Beeswax
Marshmallow Root   Oils
Marigold Flowers

Chickweed Ointment *(eczema)*

Chickweed Herb   Oils
Beeswax

BF&C Ointment *(skin, muscles)*

White Oak Bark   Skullcap Herb
Marshmallow Root   Comfrey Leaf
Mullein Herb   Black Walnut Leaf
Wormwood Herb   Gravel Root
Lobelia Herb   Olive Oil
Wheat Germ Oil   Honey

ANT-PLG *(Anti-Plague)* *(diarrhea, antimicrobial)*

Fresh Garlic   Lobelia Herb
Apple Cider Vinegar   Marshmallow Root
Vegetable Glycerine   White Oak Bark
Honey   Black Walnut Bark
Garlic Juice   Mullein Leaf
Fresh Comfrey Root   Skullcap Herb
Wormwood Herb   Uva Ursi Leaf

Colon 8 *(colon cleanser) manufactured by Ion Laboratories*

Psyllium in a base of bentonite   Goldenseal
Oat bran   Gentian
Lactobacillus acidophilus   Cascara sagrada
Whey   Aloe socotrina
Alfalfa   Calcium
Rhubarb   Magnesium
Buckthorn   Other minerals natural to the herbs

Bach Flower Essences and Rescue Remedy

Bach Flower Essences

Developed by English physician Dr. Edward Bach, Bach Flower Essences are, to the mental/emotional body, what herbs are to the physical body. The energy vibrations of the 38 flowers used in this system of healing correspond to disturbances reflected in the personality as a result of emotional distress. These disturbances can lead to physical illness. The field of psychoneuroimmunology has clearly linked emotional states of mind (such as fears, phobias, hate, anger, jealousy, low self-esteem, etc.) to physical problems. On a more esoteric level, the Essences create "internal harmony and an amplification of the higher energetic systems that connect human beings to their higher selves." (Richard Gerber, *Vibrational Medicine*, Bear & Co. 1988).

The Essences, prepared from flowers, can contribute subtle yet potent support for emotional responses to emergencies, the stress of chronic illness, or long-term conflicts within the family unit.

They can be a replacement for or an adjunct to anxiety-reducing herbs or even pharmaceutical drugs.

Rescue Remedy

The Bach formula known as Rescue Remedy is the most well known of the flower essences. It can be used in any emergency situation, great or small. It is useful, for example, upon hearing bad news, after an accident, prior to or post-surgery. It addresses issues of shock, terror, panic, mental stress, tension, confusion. Rescue Remedy's calming effect is meant to assist, not replace, medical treatment.

Rescue Remedy may be applied directly to external injuries, be used to bathe a painful area, or applied as a compress (6 drops to a pint of water).

How to Dose

- ❧ Add 4 drops of the single essence, formula of essences, or Rescue Remedy to a half glass of water, encouraging frequent sips.
- ❧ As the child grows calmer, decrease frequency and give as needed.
- ❧ If the child is unable to sip or is even unconscious, rub on the gums, lips, behind the ears, and on the wrists at intervals as frequent as every 5 minutes until emergency medical help arrives.
- ❧ Essences given for long-term conditions are given 4 times a day directly in the mouth or diluted in water.

A practitioner of Bach Flower Essences can assist in the healing of illness resulting from long-standing emotional problems by developing a formula personalized to your child.

References

The Bach Flower Essences are another tool to holistically help you support your child's body, mind, and spirit. Take charge of your child's emotional wellness. You can receive guidance in selecting appropriate remedies (there is absolutely no danger in choosing the wrong one except for having deprived your child of the right one) by reading books on the Bach Essences such as:

Handbook of the Bach Flower Remedies by Dr. Philip M.
Chancellor (Keats Publishing, 1971).
Bach Flower Remedies for Children: A Parent's Guide by Barbara
Mazzarella (Healing Arts Press, 1997)

For more information or the name of a Bach Flower practitioner near you, write to Ellon Bach U.S.A., Inc. 644 Merrick Road, Lynbrook, NY 11563 or call them at 516–593–2206.

APPENDIX J

Herbs and Their Latin Names

alfalfa *(medicago sativa)*
almond *(prunus amygdalus)*
aloe vera *(aloe vera)*
anise *(pimpinella anisum)*
arnica *(arnica montana)*
astragalus root *(astragalus membranaceous)*
barberry *(berberis vulgaris)*
bayberry *(myrica cerifera)*
black cohosh *(cimicifuga racemosa)*
black walnut *(juglans nigra)*
blessed thistle *(cnicus benedictus)*
blue cohosh *(caulophyllum thalictroides)*
boneset *(eupatorium perfoliatum)*
borage *(borago off.)*
buckthorn *(rhamnus frangula)*
burdock root *(arctium lappa)*
calendula *(calendula off.)*
cascara sagrada *(rhamnus purshiana)*
castor oil *(ricinus communis)*
catnip *(nepeta cataria)*
cayenne *(capsicum annuum)*
chamomile, German *(matricaria recutita)*
chamomile, Roman *(anthemis nobilis)*
chaparral *(larrea tridentata)*
chaste berry *(vitex agnus castus)*
chickweed *(stellaria media)*

cinnamon *(cinnamonum cassia)*
cloves *(syzygium aromaticum)*
comfrey *(symphytum off.)*
dandelion *(taraxacum off.)*
dill *(anethum graveolens)*
echinacea *(echinacea purpurea, e. angustifolia)*
elderberry *(sambucus nigra)*
eucalyptus *(eucalyptus globulus)*
evening primrose *(oenothera biennis)*
eyebright *(euphrasia off.)*
fennel *(foeniculum vulgare)*
fenugreek *(trigonella foenum-graecum)*
flaxseed *(linum usitatissimun)*
garlic *(allium sativum)*
ginger *(zingiber off.)*
ginkgo *(ginkgo biloba)*
goldenseal *(hydrastis canadensis)*
gotu kola *(centella asiatica)*
gravel root *(eupatorium purpureum)*
hops *(humulus lupulus)*
horsetail *(equisetum arvense)*
hyssop *(hyssopus off.)*
juniper berry *(juniperus communis)*
lavender oil *(lavandula off.)*
lemon balm *(melissa off.)*
lemongrass *(cymbopogon citratus)*
licorice root *(glycyrrhiza glabra)*
lobelia *(lobelia inflata)*
marshmallow root *(althea off.)*
meadowsweet *(filipendula ulmaria)*
mullein *(verbascum thapsus)*
myrrh *(commiphora molmol)*
neroli (orange blossom) *(citrus vulgaris)*
nettles *(urtica dioica)*
oak bark *(quercus alba)*
oats, oatstraw *(avena sativa)*

olive oil *(olea europaea)*
onion *(allium cepa)*
Oregon grape root *(berberis aquifolium)*
osha root *(ligusticum porteri)*
parsley *(petroselinum crispum)*
passionflower *(passiflora incarnata)*
pau d'arco *(tabebuia impetiginosa)*
pennyroyal *(mentha pulegium)*
peppermint *(mentha piperita)*
plantain *(plantago-lanceolata)*
psyllium *(plantago ovata)*
raspberry leaf *(rubus idaeus)*
red clover *(trifolium pratense)*
rosemary *(rosmarinus off.)*
sage *(salvia off.)*
sarsaparilla *(smilax off.)*
Siberian ginseng *(eleutherococcus senticosus)*
scullcap *(scutellaria lateriflora)*
slippery elm *(ulmus fulva)*
spearmint *(mentha spicata)*
St. John's Wort *(hypericum perforatum)*
tea tree *(melaleuca aternifolia)*
thyme *(thymus vulgaris)*
turkey rhubarb *(rheum palmatum)*
uva ursi *(arctostaphylos uva-ursi)*
valerian *(valeriana off.)*
white willow bark *(salix alba)*
witch hazel *(hamamelis virginiana)*
wood betony *(stachys off.)*
wormwood *(artemesia absinthium)*
yarrow *(achillea millefolium)*
yellow dock root *(rumex crispus)*

❧ Bibliography ❧

Blumenthal et al. *The Complete German Commission E Monographs*. The American Botanical Council, 1998.

Campbell, Don. *The Mozart Effect*. Avon, 1997.

Carper, Jean. *The Food Pharmacy*. Bantam, 1998.

Chancellor, Dr. Philip M. *Handbook of the Bach Flower Remedies*. Keats, 1971.

Christopher, Dr. John R. *School of Natural Healing*. Christopher Publications, 1976.

Foster, Steven, and James A. Duke. *A Field Guide to Medicinal Plants*. Houghton Mifflin, 1992.

McIntyre, Anne. *The Herbal for Mother and Child*. Element, 1992.

National Honey Board, Longmont, CO.

Wolverton, Bill. *How to Grow Fresh Air: 50 Houseplants that Purify Your Home or Office*. Penguin, 1997.

❦Index❧

gentian, 249
geranium, 166
Gerber, Richard, 250
Gilberties Herb and Garden Center, 241
ginger *(zingiber off.)*, i, 40, 57, 89–90, 91,
    128, 132, 135, 136, 137, 138, 153,
    170, 194, 200, 221, 247, 248
ginkgo *(ginkgo biloba)*, 182
glands, swollen, 77–78, 113
glycerine, 165, 248, 249
goldenseal *(hydrastis canadensis)*, 61, 69,
    76, 84, 124, 125, 201, 220, 247, 248,
    249
gotu kola *(centella asiatica)*, 183
grains, 82, 169, 192, 231
    See also specific grains
grapefruit seed extract, 60–61
grapes, grapeseed oil, 71, 90, 147, 184,
    232
gravel root *(eupatorium purpureum)*, 31,
    248, 249
gums, inflamed, 81, 83–84, 158

Handbook of the Bach Flower Remedies
    (Chancellor), 251
hands, warm, 128
Hanna's Herb Shop, 140, 241
Harvard Medical School, 8, 130
hay fever, 56, 202, 205, 206, 247
headaches, 56, 57, 58, 70–75, 169, 170,
    187, 203, 209, 214, 235, 236, 238
Healers Who Share, 52, 243
Healing Into Immortality (Epstein), 32
Healing Power of Herbs (TV show), 92
Healing Visualizations (Epstein), 32, 235
hearing impairment, 62, 66
heartburn, 141–44
heart problems, 221
heat rash, prickly, 120
Herbal Eyebright formula, 69, 205, 248
Herbalgram, 244
herbalist, master, 243
Herb Research Foundation, The, 244
herbs
    administering, 14–15, 36–37, 50, 53
    characteristics of, 219–21
    encapsulated, 69, 168–69, 213–14, 216
    soothing, 18–19, 22–23, 25–30, 31, 35,
        44–48, 61, 70, 73, 81, 87, 93, 94,
        110, 113–14, 124, 137, 146, 154,
        155, 220
    sources of, 216–18

storing and preserving, 216
symposia of, 245
vaporizing, 201–2
    See also dosing; *specific herbs*
Heritage Products, 115, 242
hernia, hiatal, 142
herpes virus, 82
hiccoughs, 139–40
Hippocrates, 19, 135
hives, 109–10, 203, 204–5
Holistic Resource Network Directory,
    The, 244
Homeopathic Educational Services,
    238
homeopathy, 239, 240, 241, 243–44
    for adrenal glands, 103
    for anaphylaxis, 49–50
    for asthma, 105–6
    for Lyme disease, 52
    for nerves, 207
    for pain, 36, 40
    for poison ivy, 53–54
    and vaccinations, 159, 160
    *See also specific cell salts; specific
        homeopathic remedies*
Honegar, 106, 132, 161–62, 163
honey, i, 14, 19–20, 25–26, 48, 61, 70, 71,
    77, 78, 80, 86–87, 92, 105, 106, 121,
    131, 132, 134, 154, 162, 165, 177,
    178, 185, 191, 193, 194, 205–6, 210,
    232, 249
hops *(humulus lupulus)*, 38, 40, 58, 73,
    103, 179, 202, 221, 247
horsetail *(equisetum arvense)*, 32, 185
hot flashes, 133
How to Grow Fresh Air (Wolverton), 99
hydration. *See* fluids
hydrogen peroxide, 11, 20
hyssop *(hyssopus off.)*, 79, 90

imagery, healing, 32, 74–75, 102, 178,
    234–37
immune system, i, 51–52, 56, 62–63, 79,
    82, 91, 92, 100, 104, 107, 113, 115,
    125, 127, 148, 157, 159, 171, 182,
    187, 190–210, 228, 235, 238
impetigo, 125
infection, 16, 23, 38, 57, 92, 94, 97, 104,
    113, 115–17, 122–23, 132, 153, 155,
    157, 158, 191, 199, 203, 209, 214,
    230
    See also specific infections

wheat germ oil, 25, 26, 29, 249
wheezing, 104, 105, 106
whey, 249
white oak bark. *See* oak bark
white willow bark *(salix alba)*, 36, 37, 39, 160
wild oats. *See* oats, oatstraw
wild yam root, 137, 220
witch hazel *(hamamelis virginiana)*, 37
Wolverton, Bill, 99
Wolverton Environmental Services, 100
Woman's Book of Life, A (Borysenko), 172
wood betony *(stachys off.)*, 247
World Health Organization (WHO), 2
worms, 140–41
wormwood *(artemesia absinthium)*, 31, 221, 248, 249

wounds, 18–24, 56, 115–17, 235
www.holistic-resource.com, 244
www.Mozarteffect.com, 187
www.naturopathic.org, 243

yarrow *(achillea millefolium)*, 74, 79, 157, 200, 201, 219, 232
yeast, 66, 146, 147–48, 153, 186, 208–10, 231
yellow dock root *(rumex crispus)*, 119, 123
yoga, 42, 177
yogurt, 12–13, 28, 64, 71, 114, 131, 133, 134, 135, 148, 154, 191, 214

zinc, 26, 166

Printed in the United States
By Bookmasters